WHY AM I SO TIRED?

Why am I so Tired?

Is Your Thyroid Making you Ill?

MARTIN BUDD N.D., D.O.

Thorsons

Thorsons
An Imprint of HarperCollins*Publishers*
77–85 Fulham Palace Road,
Hammersmith, London W6 8JB

The Thorsons website address is: www.thorsons.com

Published by Thorsons 2000

9 10 8

A catalogue record for this book
is available from the British Library

ISBN 0 7225 3942 8

Printed and bound in Great Britain by
Martins the Printers Ltd, Berwick upon Tweed

Contents

Acknowledgement

This book could not have been written without the enthusiastic support of my wife, Maggie.

By the same author:

Low Blood Sugar
Diets to Help Diabetes
Diets to Help Migraine
Recipes for Health: Low Blood Sugar (with Maggie Budd)

Introduction

My interest in low grade or mild hypothyroidism began in the early 1980s. Following the publication of my first book *Low Blood Sugar* (hypoglycaemia) in 1981, I was consulted by many exhausted, depressed patients who having read the book were convinced that they had discovered the mystery cause behind their symptoms. However, it soon became apparent to me as I became more familiar with the diagnosis of hypoglycaemia, that approximately one third of the patients did not suffer from low blood sugar, but their fatigue was caused by another illness – undiagnosed mild hypothyroidism.

Hypothyroidism is often missed in patients suffering from fatigue because many of these people do not fit into the medical definition of 'hypothyroid'; many hypothyroid patients show clear test results under the accepted medical blood tests or do not fit into the typical picture of an overweight, middle-aged hypothyroid sufferer. For example, many young hypothyroid patients are not overweight but underweight. Men and women of all ages can develop thyroid problems, and there are over 100 symptoms caused by thyroid deficiency. The overweight middle-aged female with exhaustion and alopecia may well be the archetypal patient but a 'typical' thyroid syndrome does not exist. ***Each patient can present their own unique symptom*** *picture.* Every organ and system in the body can be disturbed when the thyroid is underactive, and a mild thyroid malfunction can give rise to 10–20 different symptoms in each patient. Symptoms as diverse as leg cramps, allergic rhinitis, constipation, period pains and poor memory have all been attributed to hypothyroidism.

Mild or early stage health problems often go undiagnosed as laboratory tests identify only major blood changes. This has led to a situation where many suffer symptoms of illness – but not 'clinically' bad enough for a blood test diagnosis to be made.

Blood tests are only a reliable guide to diagnosis when the procedures for testing and the interpretation of the results are standardized. For example, with the diagnosis of diabetes, the test procedures and the normal ranges for blood glucose are internationally recognized. The test results therefore provide a reliable guide to the diagnosis, the severity and the successful treatment of diabetes. Unfortunately, the same cannot be said when testing for thyroid disorders.

In *Why am I so Tired?* I discuss many of the symptoms, treatments and causes of this underdiagnosed health condition. In Part One I describe how the thyroid influences the body and explain in detail the most common symptoms of untreated hypothyroidism. In Part Two I compare and elucidate the different diagnostic methods and show you some simple diagnostic tests you can carry out easily at home. I discuss both medical and naturopathic treatment and illustrate how diet, exercise and lifestyle changes, can go a long way to relieving your symptoms. Lastly, I discuss many of the underlying causes of a thyroid disorder so you can not only treat your symptoms more effectively, but learn to understand how your body became fatigued. I also discuss some of the different causes and diagnostic techniques for fatigue itself, so that you may begin to treat fatigue even if you feel hypothyroidism may not be the underlying illness.

I hope that with the help of this book you can begin to fight your fatigue and recover your natural health, energy and vitality.

PART ONE

Fatigue and weariness can slowly take over your body. You may find it difficult to motivate yourself, to become excited or express enthusiasm; body and mind are slow and heavy. Some of you may be painfully aware of this change in energy level, others may have experienced tiredness for so long it seems natural and cannot remember a time they felt vital or energetic ... if ever.

However, with the guidance of this book you can return to health. Here is the success story of one woman I helped through fatigue, stress and depression to finally recognize and treat her undiagnosed mild hypothyroidism.

Liz's Story

Liz had felt exhausted for four years. Prior to her total hysterectomy four and a half years ago, she had been a slim, active mother in her early forties with two teenage children and the happy wife of a successful caring husband.

She had hoped that after her hysterectomy she would enjoy a future without the monthly burden of heavy, painful periods caused by endometriosis. However, after three months convalescence, she felt certain that in her own words – 'something was wrong'. Within six months of the operation, Liz looked a different person. She was 20lb over her normal weight of 125lb, and her usual robust colour was replaced by an unhealthy pallor with dark shadows beneath her eyes. All of which made her look 10 years older than her 46 years. Although Liz was concerned about her looks, she was far more worried about how she felt.

The Tiredness

We all feel tired – or fatigued – now and again. Usually we can put it down to a few too many late nights, or maybe an unexpected stress or illness, maybe even just working too hard. This transient fatigue lifts after a few early nights or a restful holiday. Unfortunately the type of chronic fatigue you might be experiencing does not go away. You may *constantly* feel tired, your body may feel heavy all the time and simply concentrating on your work or completing the household chores may take all the energy you have. You – like Liz – may be suffering from a type of fatigue which cannot be solved by early nights or a holiday. Liz realized that her energy levels and work capacity compared very unfavourably with her pre-hysterectomy vitality; although, you may not be able to pin down your exhaustion to a single event or cause, you probably realize that you are not your normal, energetic, and happy self.

Liz ached with fatigue. Her neck, shoulders and lower back were stiff and painful. Her hands and feet were always cold and occasionally numb, and dull frontal headaches had become a daily pattern. Far from sleep refreshing her, she felt worse on waking and claimed that she 'didn't really surface until mid-day'. The physical exhaustion was accompanied by mental exhaustion, this caused her to feel depressed. Her increasingly poor concentration and memory were the cause of many problems. Although she could remember her childhood with some clarity, her short-term memory was unreliable. She frequently lost her car keys and shopping lists, and missed appointments. On several occasions she could not recall where her car was parked and was obliged to take a taxi home.

The Domestic Stress

For Liz everything was an effort, she felt drained, confused and unhappy. Her exhaustion and depression lead to frustration, irritability, and anxiety. Her husband Mike, found that his business as a garden designer begun to suffer. Liz had looked after his books and accounts for many years, but now her poor concentration and moodiness resulted in lost and dissatisfied clients. Arguments between Liz and her husband became daily events. We can all absorb stress from our partners, and certainly Mike was becoming anxious and increasingly baffled by his wife's attitude and behaviour.

Their marriage was not helped by Liz's loss of interest in sex. The sexual side of their partnership had always been mutually satisfying and relaxing, but for Liz this had lapsed under the familiar excuse of 'too much effort'. For the same reason Liz felt unable to continue the dancing and golf that they had both enjoyed for many years. Mike had complained to his doctor that he thought the hysterectomy had changed his wife's personality. By the time Liz consulted me her weight had risen to 170lb, being 45lb over her ideal weight.

In addition to her exhaustion and other symptoms, Liz complained that if she did not eat every two or three hours she would tremble and feel dizzy and breathless, and often experienced a sugar craving. Because of this she had increased her meal frequency to include snacks of sugar-rich pastries and drinks. This new habit, coupled with her lack of exercise and general sluggishness, served to further increase her weight.

After four years of ill health, Liz had become trapped in a vicious circle of exhaustion, depression, obesity and anxiety. Her natural optimism and self-esteem were at zero.

When Liz discussed her symptoms with her doctor a few months after her operation, she was told that she was simply suffering the after effects of major surgery, and the consequences of an overnight menopause. He requested a blood screen including full biochemistry, haematology and thyroid profiles. The only test 'out of range' was a slightly raised cholesterol. There was no evidence of anaemia and *the thyroid hormone levels appeared normal*. Liz was told that her blood pressure was also normal, but she was advised to lose weight by reducing the fat and sugar in her diet. She was prescribed a low dose HRT and an antidepressant. Unfortunately after trying several antidepressants and attempting unsuccessfully to diet, Liz was still overweight, depressed and exhausted. Moreover, she was confused, the doctor had said her tests were 'normal' and yet she felt far from her 'normal' self.

MY DIAGNOSIS

Although the thyroid test showed results within the medically-defined normal range, I considered that Liz had many symptoms that one could attribute to a low grade or mildly underactive thyroid. I therefore requested another thyroid profile (her last test being four years earlier), and instructed her to test her morning temperatures (see pages 127-30) for three consecutive days.

The blood test showed a blood thyroxine to be at the lower end of the normal range. The average morning temperature was 96.8°F (36°C) (the normal range is between 97.8°F [36.6°C] and 98.2°F [36.8°C]).

THE TREATMENT

The combination of a borderline blood test result, a low morning temperature and her symptoms confirmed for me that Liz was suffering from mild hypothyroidism. She was advised to follow a suitable diet and to take nutritional supplements to support the thyroid. Thyroid extract (animal thyroid) in tablet form was also prescribed. Liz began to show symptom-relief and reduced depression within six weeks.

After three months of treatment her blood test showed an improvement. Her average basal morning temperatures rose to 97.2°F (36.2°C).

After six months of treatment Liz's weight was 135lb and her energy was much improved. Other symptoms including the headaches, muscle stiffness, pain and poor concentration were all at least 50 per cent better. The depression had cleared and Liz had stopped taking the anti-depressants.

Does this story strike a chord with you? Do you feel constantly tired, depressed and confused? Do you find it difficult to explain why you feel exhausted all the time – and maybe have even forgotten what it is like NOT to feel tired?

These feelings are common emotions for a sufferer of hypothyroidism.

CHAPTER ONE

'What is the Thyroid?'

The Thyroid Gland and Your Body

Most of us have read or heard about the thyroid gland and have some idea of what it does in the body. However, few of us have a completely accurate picture of the thyroid and if asked what function it holds in our bodies, would simply reply: 'It controls our metabolism. Overweight people have slow metabolisms, slim people have faster metabolisms.'

However, there is a lot more to the thyroid than weight or energy. In fact, your thyroid can be compared to the choke on your car: increased fuel increases engine revs, while decreased fuel reduces the revs. Consequently, if your choke does not work properly the rest of your body will suffer. You will feel slow, lethargic and find it impossible to get going in the mornings.

Indeed, the thyroid does regulate our metabolism, but this does not merely influence our weight, it also directly controls oxygen turnover in every cell in the body as well as temperature control and hormones. Our hormones direct nearly every system or process in the body, including: growth, energy, sex drive, circulatory efficiency, muscle and joint flexibility and immune efficiency. Our entire blood supply – approximately 10 pints – circulates through the thyroid gland once every 60 minutes.

The thyroid gland has a mental, as well as physical role. Our brains are influenced by a decline in our metabolic rate and symptoms similar to premature ageing can develop, including: poor short-term memory, mental fatigue, difficulty in concentrating, anxiety and moodiness. Therefore, you can see that if our thyroid is not working efficiently we may experience a whole range of different symptoms!

Where is it Located?

Your thyroid gland lies at the front of your neck, between your breastbone and Adam's apple. The gland lies across your windpipe and has a butterfly-like appearance; two lobes are joined by a narrow band of tissue known as an 'isthmus'.

You can palpate your own thyroid gland by stretching your neck and pulling your head back. If you then swallow you may see or feel the gland rise and fall. Not all of us can see or palpate our thyroid, so do not be concerned if this exercise does not work. Men's thyroids can usually be located more easily than women's.

How Large is it?

There is considerable variation in the size and weight of the thyroid. The weight can vary from 8g to 40g. It is also possible to be born without a thyroid gland (this is called cretinism). Thyroid tissue can exist and function some distance from the main gland, this aberrant or anomalous tissue – coupled with the great range in size and weight – demonstrates that there is no standard thyroid gland.

What is 'Hypothyroidism'?

In some people, the thyroid gland does not work correctly and this can be due to any number of causes (see Appendix A). When the thyroid does not work as hard as it should and becomes 'underactive' the patient is diagnosed with 'hypothyroidism', ('hypo' is Greek for 'under'). Hypothyroidism can also be called 'myxoedema'. This term is used in more severe cases of hypothyroidism and refers to a type of body swelling which can occur. 'Euthyroidism' means a normal thyroid and 'hyperthyroidism' refers to an overactive thyroid.

> Around 10 per cent of the adult population of Great Britain suffer symptoms caused by mild hypothyroidism. American doctors and researchers have put the figure in the US even higher.

As I have mentioned, when the gland becomes underactive every aspect of our metabolism is acted upon and the levels of water, proteins, fats and cholesterol all increase. Therefore, the functions mentioned above – including temperature, immunity, energy, growth, sex drive, memory – are all adversely affected and usually decrease.

> It is quite incorrect to say that hypothyroidism is a female complaint. Approximately 10 per cent of the 300 thyroid patients that I have treated over the last four years have been men. Although the majority of my patients are in the over-fifty range, I have treated teenagers with a diagnosis of mild hypothyroidism, who have responded well to the appropriate treatment.

One of the commonest symptoms of an underactive thyroid – and one which greatly concerns us – is tiredness or fatigue. This is a result of the slowing down of all the body's systems and organs.

Many patients with an underactive thyroid gland comment that they 'wake up some time after their eyes are open!'. The thyroid is the body's internal clock and when the gland is inefficient or underactive the metabolism does not usually recover from the effects of sleep until around mid-day.

The Thyroid Hormones

The thyroid gland releases two hormones which in turn influence virtually every cell in the body. These two essential hormones are **thyroxine** (T_4) and **triiodothyronine** (T_3). The T_4 and T_3 denotes the number of iodine atoms in the hormone molecules, iodine being the chief constituent of the thyroid hormones.

Only T_3 is chemically active at cell level, the non-active T_4 is converted to T_3 only when required. There exists around 50 times more T_4 than T_3 in the blood, and the two hormones are linked to, and transported in the blood by carrier proteins. It is only when the hormones are free of the protein (at which time they are measured in the blood as free T_4 and free T_3) that they become chemically active.

The thyroid is controlled by the pituitary gland. The pituitary responds to a low level of blood thyroid hormones by releasing thyroid stimulating hormone (TSH).

The pituitary gland is under the control of the hypothalamus. This part of the brain releases thyrotrophin releasing hormone (TRH) which regulates pituitary activity.

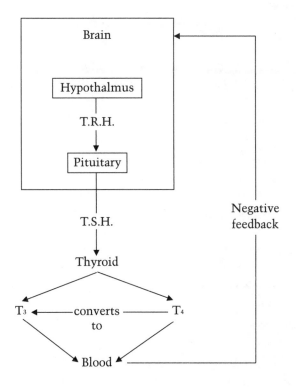

Figure 1: Thyroid control

Calcitonin

This hormone is also released by the thyroid. Its function is to regulate the blood level of calcium by reducing excessively high levels.

What are the Symptoms of Hypothyroidism?

As the thyroid influences every system, organ and muscle in the body, the potential list of symptoms is enormous. The pattern of symptoms a sufferer may experience depends on human individuality, which results from heredity, diet, immune efficiency and stress levels. Our genetic predisposition also plays an important role in influencing the systems and organs that may be disturbed by a thyroid deficiency.

However, there are certain leading symptoms that are common to the greater majority of patients, these are included in the table below.

Common symptoms of hypothyroidism

Endocrine (hormonal and glandular)	Digestive	Respiratory	Heart and circulation
Irregular periods	Thrush	Congestion	Palpitations
Painful periods	Loss of appetite	Chest infections	High blood pressure
Light periods	Irritable bowel syndrome		Hypoglycaemia
PMS	Constipation		Chilblains and bruising
Reduced libido			Cramp when walking

Skin/Hair/Nails	Muscles/Joints	Ear/Nose/Throat	Kidney/Bladder
Poor wound healing	Fibromyalgia	Hearing loss	Cystitis
Reduced perspiration	Carpal tunnel syndrome	Poor night vision	Bladder frequency

Coldness	Osteoporosis	Sinus infections
Eczema/psoriasis		Tinnitus
/acne	Shoulder/neck pain	
Dull hair	Cracking joints	

Nervous system	Miscellaneous symptoms
Poor memory	Fatigue
Mental confusion	Insomnia
Depression	Weight increase/decrease
Poor reflexes	Slow growth in children
Poor concentration	Headaches

How is Hypothyroidism Tested?

Modern blood testing is seen as an essential component in diagnosing hypothyroidism. Doctors measure the amount of thyroxine (T4) and triiodothyronine (T3) to assess how well the gland is working. (They also measure free T4 and free T3.) Many doctors and researchers also measure the amount of TSH or thyrotropin in your blood stream. TSH is released when there is too little T4 so the more TSH you have in your body the more underactive your thyroid (and the less TSH the more overactive your thyroid).

However, blood testing is a controversial method of testing for hypothyroidism as many people experience the symptoms of low grade hypothyroidism, yet show apparently normal blood test results. Moreover, many sufferers do not fit into the medical catagories doctors expect. For example, many young hypothyroid patients are not overweight, but are often underweight. Despite the fact that the majority of patients being treated for hypothyroidism by the medical profession fall into a broad 'overweight middle-aged female' category, men and women of all ages can develop thyroid problems at any time in their life. As there are over 100 symptoms caused by thyroid deficiency each patient can show a unique combination of symptoms; even a case of mild hypothyroidism can give rise to between 10 and 20 different symptoms in each patient.

Blood test results are created by comparing the patient's amount of thyroxine, triiodothyronine and TSH against standard test ranges. However, the normal ranges do not always reflect what is optimum for the patient.

In order to explain this clearly let's look at a fictitious Helen. If Helen has a thyroxine (free T4) level of 12, this would be seen by her practitioner as normal. (The medical standard range for a normal level of thyroxine is between 10 and 25.) However, for Helen to feel healthy and well her optimum level of thyroxine should be 18. This means that her test may meet the medical standard but it is still too low *for her.* Consequently, Helen continues to suffer from the diverse symptoms of hypothyroidism even though her GP has told her that everything is normal and she does not have a thyroid malfunction.

The only reliable method to assess and understand the 'normal' levels of thyroid hormones for each patient is to request blood thyroid profiles when they are symptom free. This is rarely done. Thyroid testing is not usually required for insurance examinations and healthy patients do not normally request blood tests. I believe that apart from severe thyroid disease, blood test evidence is only of value in thyroid diagnosis when used in conjunction with the elements mentioned below.

As there is no archetypal patient with 'typical symptoms' and the modern blood test is unreliable, many people suffer needlessly from hypothyroid symptoms. If you feel you may be suffering from a mildly underactive thyroid it is important to base any diagnosis on three elements:

1   Morning temperatures
2   Symptom assessment
3   Blood test results

In Part Two of this book I will show you how to use each of these elements accurately and safely (in conjunction with a health practitioner) so that you can begin to recover from your mild hypothyroidism.

CHAPTER TWO

'Why do I Feel so Tired?'

The Thyroid Gland and Your Fatigue

'Why am I so tired?' is a question many of you may have asked your doctor or health practitioner. We all feel tired after exercise or a hard day at work – but the constant exhaustion which may lead you to consult a professional is entirely different. This type of tiredness is all-consuming. You may feel completely drained no matter how little physical or mental effort you may have made during the day. You do not even feel better after a good night's sleep, in fact you may feel worse. This constant fatigue may leave you depressed and anxious, it occupies your mind and embraces your body leaving you confused as to what is wrong with you.

Fatigue is the second commonest symptom that affects mankind – the commonest symptom being pain – and is also the most frequent symptom of mild hypothyroidism. As outlined in this book, the diagnosis and treatment of this frequently missed problem is an important first step in treating many very tired patients.

Fatigue itself cannot be treated effectively. In fact any attempt to rev up the body's energy production is usually doomed to failure. Vitamin and mineral injections and nutritional tonics may be temporarily supportive, but for lasting relief it is essential to uncover and treat the cause, or causes, of your fatigue.

How Does the Thyroid Cause Fatigue?

The link between thyroid malfunction and fatigue is well recognized by practitioners and patients. However, it may interest you to know just how a tiny gland weighing between 8gm and 40gm (or less than 2oz) can profoundly influence all our systems and organs.

The patterns of cause and effect with the thyroid and fatigue are both subtle and complex. Many of the symptoms that develop as a result of a thyroid imbalance contribute to the condition and a vicious circle is established. These symptoms include obesity (causing reduced activity), depression, muscle pain and sugar cravings.

In order to explain your fatigue, we first need to define 'fatigue' itself: What is it? Can it be measured? And how do we know when we are tired?

Measuring Your Fatigue

For a variety of reasons, fatigue is difficult to recognize, measure and treat. Perhaps the main cause of this difficulty is the nature of the symptom. Fatigue is essentially a subjective symptom. Subjective meaning, 'due to internal causes and discoverable by oneself alone'. It is a symptom that can be easily masked, you can put on make-up or feign jollity. Therefore, unlike many other symptoms, your fatigue is not always obvious to other people.

Measuring fatigue is another challenge. There are very few health problems that cause a predictable level of fatigue. One immediately thinks of anaemia, the exhaustion of terminal illness or chronic insomnia. Yet I have known patients who were seriously ill with cancer, yet were able to draw on diminishing reserves and present a deceptively normal, even lively demeanour. Our level of fatigue can vary almost from hour to hour, for many factors influence our energy levels. These factors include our blood sugar status, our mood, current and past stress, infection, occupation, how we sleep and for women, the monthly pattern determined by the female hormones. Not forgetting the 30 to 40 illnesses that feature fatigue as a major, predictable symptom. Our state of mind often influences our apparent state of fatigue. How often do we experience an energy surge when receiving good news or meeting a friend or partner?

So as I have said, fatigue is not easy to recognize or to measure in ourselves or in others. Our level of health and any symptoms experienced are unique to each of us. However, in order to tell if you may be fatigued, you can start by asking yourself three simple questions:

1   **How do you know you are tired?**
2   **Do you remember a time in the past when you were not tired?**
3   **Have you compared your energy levels with colleagues, friends or family members?**

The answer to the first question usually leads on to the other two questions. This is because our assessment of how tired we are is usually based on comparison with how we have felt in the past, or comparisons with those who we know and regularly meet.

Typical answers you might reply include:

'I know I am much more tired than I was six months ago'
'I am always the first in our group to want to go home or go to bed'

More often than not, if you suffer with chronic or long-term fatigue you may have forgotten what it is like to feel normal. You have been tired for so long that you have no memory of better, more vital times. This lack of awareness of the severity of your problem presents a challenge to a practitioner, simply because you can only compare your state of health with friends and family around you. You have therefore lost the potentially more reliable and accurate comparison based on how you yourself once felt.

Consequently, when attempting to assess your fatigue levels, you will find it of great value to talk to your partner or a close relative. Not surprisingly fatigue can influence our mood, our lifestyle and our activities. It is often those close to us who notice changes in our behaviour.

Fatigue can also influence how we look. A loss of sparkle in the eyes, grey outlines beneath the eyes and a postural slump, are all give-away clues to chronic fatigue.

Laboratory Measurements for Fatigue

Health practitioners use laboratory tests to measure if you are fatigued. This is an essential first step to recovery (see chapter nine).

I am quite frequently consulted by fatigued patients who have been offered a diagnosis of chronic fatigue syndrome, fibromyalgia or depression, yet without the evidence of blood and other laboratory tests. I believe it is wise to eliminate the obvious reasons for fatigue before worrying about more obscure illnesses. Certainly late-onset diabetes, pernicious anaemia and nutritional deficiencies need to be considered in elderly patients. Likewise iron deficient anaemia, hypoglycaemia and the effects of stress need to be investigated in young and middle-aged patients.

Tests a doctor or practitioner may offer you can include:

* An assessment of blood fats, kidney, gall bladder and liver function, proteins and blood glucose.
* A haematology profile. This test measures the red and white cells in the blood, assesses iron transport, inflammation, and

the clotting factor. A differential count of the white cells also offers information on the immune system.

* A mineral profile. This involves your practitioner taking a sample of hair, blood, sweat or urine.
* A full thyroid profile is also requested to assess if you may be tired.
* A temperature check.
* A six-hour glucose tolerance test may also be needed.
* A red cell essential fatty acid profile may be of value. This measures the blood levels of the omega 3 and 6 series and other fatty acids.
* Occasionally, where indicated, a urine amino acid investigation may be requested.

One needs to be selective when requesting tests. There are over one thousand tests in current use, so it is important for the practitioner to tailor the tests to the patient. If this is not done a lot of money, time, and perhaps patient rapport can be wasted or lost. My procedure for testing for fatigue is described in chapter 11.

PEGGY'S STORY

I had known and treated Peggy, who was a very active 85 year old widow, for 16 years. She had always taken care of herself, eating well and avoiding cigarettes and excessive alcohol. She had suffered a tendency to be overweight, although her blood pressure was always normal. Knee and lower back stiffness and pain, particularly in the winter, and a slightly raised cholesterol had all needed treatment. None of these problems however had caused her great concern and she freely admitted that her motivation to consult me was entirely based on her love of golf. She played two half rounds each week, which provided her with exercise, and what she termed 'a healthy challenge'. She also met her friends and enjoyed a pleasant social lunch at the club house. She saw her visits to my surgery as necessary maintenance to enable her to continue her one sporting activity, around which her social life revolved.

Peggy's concern began when she found that her stamina only allowed her to complete two or three holes. This had developed very slowly over a six month period. Routine cardiovascular checks were carried out by her doctor, but nothing was discovered except for the slightly raised cholesterol and a raised uric acid (this was in line with the fact Peggy suffered from mild gout).

Her doctor further requested a bone density scan to assess osteoporosis risk and a full biochemistry and haematology screen. No other imbalances or deficiencies showed. He made it clear to Peggy that at her age she should now discontinue golf and settle for the occasional short walk. He also advised her to lose weight and avoid the foods and drinks that can lead to gout.

She was not happy with her doctor's diagnosis and even less happy with his recommended treatment.

After Peggy had reassured me that she was sleeping well and that she had not suffered recent infections or stress, I questioned her for more detailed information on her fatigue. She was able to confirm my suspicions that she was also suffering mental fatigue, described by her as a 'mental fog'. This included poor memory and concentration, and a reduced sense of smell and taste. Peggy also remarked that her hands and feet had been unusually cold over the previous few months.

I requested a morning temperature check and thyroid blood tests. In addition I asked the laboratory to check Peggy's levels of minerals and vitamin B^{12}.

> Vitamin B$_{12}$ absorption is reduced with hypothyroidism. Lack of this vitamin in humans can cause fatigue, neuralgia, poor memory and general sluggish thinking.
>
> In common with many other nutrients, it cannot be assumed that eating a good diet offers sufficient protection from deficiencies. Food digestion and absorption depends on many interactions, nutrients and enzymes.

Peggy's morning temperatures showed an average of 96.8°F (36°C). Her vitamin B$_{12}$ and thyroid hormones were all within the normal ranges, but towards the lower end of each range. Her minerals showed deficiencies in magnesium, zinc, chromium and manganese.

TREATMENT

Peggy was prescribed a course of weekly vitamin B$_{12}$ injections, a suitable multi-mineral, and a thyroid glandular supplement.

After the third week she began to feel less fatigued and after three months of treatment she was more mentally alert and had returned to her 18 holes of golf each week. It may be necessary for Peggy to continue with the thyroid and mineral support on a low maintenance dosage for the rest of her life, coupled with monthly B$_{12}$ injections.

Maintenance treatment is often justified and worthwhile to maintain necessary health and morale in the elderly. I firmly believe that the elderly benefit from regular gentle exercise. The value of rest can be overstated, as inactivity can cause joint stiffness, muscle weakening and excess weight. Exercise also improves bone health and reduces the risk of osteoporosis.

FATIGUE – OTHER NAMES

It may be helpful to discuss the various medical titles that have been used in the UK and the USA to define chronic exhaustion.

Myalgic Encephalomyelitis (ME)

This grand sounding name is synonymous with post viral fatigue (PVF) and also interchangeable with chronic fatigue syndrome (CFS) and fibromyalgia syndrome (FMS). Past definitions for ME have included epidemic neurasthenia, Epstein-Barr syndrome, Royal Free disease and Icelandic disease. The symptoms of ME have also been defined by the media as 'Yuppy 'Flu' or chronic influenza. The chief symptom of ME is chronic fatigue, of a type that requires bedrest but offers little clinical evidence with testing. A history of recurring infections, headaches and muscle pains are characteristic. Observable signs can include throat inflammation and lymph node enlargement in the neck and armpits.

In the US, ME is usually defined as CFS or chronic fatigue and immune dysfunction syndrome (CFIDS). The criteria for diagnosis are similar to ME and many doctors believe that the simple definition CFS will become the internationally recognized title for chronic fatigue.

Post-Viral Fatigue (PVF)

By definition this title describes the chronic fatigue that follows a virus infection. There is usually a history of a viral illness (e.g. Epstein-Barr virus, glandular fever or influenza). The signs are similar to ME and involve lymph node swelling and tenderness. PVF usually shows a history of fever. However, many doctors and researchers have recorded low body temperatures with their ME and PVF patients.

Fibromyalgia

Once known as fibrositis, fibromyalgia like ME and PVS, is often seen as being under the CFS umbrella. The only slight difference being that fibromyalgia patients have mainly muscle-joint symptoms with fatigue, while ME or PVF patients exhibit more symptoms of immune system weakness coupled with their fatigue.

Hyperventilation Syndrome (HV)

Breathing difficulties linked with anxiety and spinal health are found as a common component of fibromyalgia. However, HV is generally seen as a symptom not a cause. It is appropriate to quote Leon Chaitow who has written: 'After some 15 years of treating fatigue problems and over 30 years of treating musculoskeletal pain problems, I can categorically state that I have seldom, if ever, failed to find at least "some" degree of breathing dysfunction in people with chronic fatigue syndrome (ME) or fibromyalgia.'[1]

Gulf War Syndrome

Soldiers and other personnel who were involved in the Gulf War have subsequently suffered from chronic fatigue amongst other symptoms. The cause is thought to be a combination of immunization side effects, the toxic atmospheric pollution, poor hygiene, various toxic sprays, and stress. Although these victims of the war are relatively few (30,000 plus), what happened in the Gulf may encourage a greater willingness by the medical establishments to consider environmental and chemical factors when diagnosing chronic fatigue.

The Problems of Diagnosis

Many people suffering from chronic fatigue do not fit into a neat medical pigeon hole. This situation has unfortunately lead some medical doctors to define chronic fatigue as psychosomatic (mind–body). This diagnosis is often followed with a prescription for drugs to treat anxiety and/or depression.

There may be no evidence of disease or damage with fatigue, but there is often evidence of malfunction. Functional medicine recognizes that the simple under-efficiency of a gland, organ or system, can give rise to symptoms. Nowhere is this more clearly shown than in mild or low grade hypothyroidism. This concept of imbalance or mild hypofunction rarely applies to a single function. The domino effect often applies to ill health.

> The concept of several poorly functioning but non-diseased glands has been termed multiple enzyme deficiency syndrome (MED), polyendocrine syndrome (PS) or polyendocrinopathy.

An underactive thyroid can lead to adrenal exhaustion, muscle pain, fatigue, obesity, depression and a host of other symptoms. With many health problems there exist recognizable degrees of severity. This can be seen very clearly in diabetic patients. The diagnosis of diabetes can range from a mild glucose intolerance in old age needing care with carbohydrate foods, to a severe diabetic requiring three or four insulin injections daily to stay alive. This concept of 'shades of grey' can be applied to almost any illness. Unfortunately a certain standardization of definitions is required in order to determine drug dosages and treatment protocol, so many conditions are diagnosed in terms of 'black or white'. Hypothyroidism is seen as either severe enough to warrant a lifelong prescription for thyroxine or normal and no treatment is offered.

Functional assessment requires a more sensitive awareness of test results based on a full knowledge of the patients symptoms. Unfortunately many British GPs are simply given a patient's test results, stating 'normal'. Yet it is the GP who is in contact with the patient, not the laboratory staff. The diagnosis of mild or early-stage imbalances can easily be missed with this method. The need for more sensitive tests to assess disorders of function, and mild deficiencies or excesses, has lead in the last 10 years to the development of a range of specific laboratory tests. These have included tests to measure or identify leaky gut, malabsorption, candidiasis, gut transit speed, stomach emptying speed, pancreatic enzyme status, 24-hour adrenal function tests and many more.

Therefore the key to understanding the reasons for your fatigue consists of careful test selection and subsequent test interpretation. When this is carried out efficiently and assessed alongside the symptoms you may feel, some understanding of your problem can be achieved and an accurate diagnosis arrived at. Although changes to diet and supplement use are usually harmless, the good response to any treatment depends on specificity (see page 148). The correct supplements and dosages and the appropriate food and drink are always preferable to guesswork. Once you have drawn together a symptom picture as shown in Part Two, and armed with the results of your practitioner's tests, you can begin to recover from your tiredness and enjoy renewed vitality and well-being.

CHAPTER THREE

'Why Can't I Lose Weight?'

The Thyroid Gland and Your Weight

JANE'S STORY

Jane had battled with her weight since her early teens, when she consulted me she had peaked at 174lb. With her height at 5ft her ideal weight was 120–130lb.

THE CONSULTATION

At her initial consultation Jane was aged 27 years, and in spite of a careful diet she had increased her weight by 5–6lb a month over the previous six months. Prior to this Jane had always been a lively, happy young woman with a settled job in the family business and a caring fiancé. She was concerned that the recent weight increase was making her ill, for she now suffered from fatigue, depression and low backache. Her doctor and her family were convinced that her increasing weight (now 50lb over her optimum weight) was causing the backache and fatigue, and these symptoms were making her depressed.

I know from my many years in practice that being overweight does not inevitably cause fatigue and depression, having encountered many underweight exhausted patients, and many overweight patients who were happy and full of energy.

Jane had also linked the fatigue to her weight, because the fatigue and depression had developed when her weight suddenly increased eight months previously, and her doctor's comments had endorsed her suspicions.

Everyone including Jane believed that all her symptoms would improve if she could only lose 50lb of her surplus weight.

Unfortunately, the low fat diet that she usually followed to control her weight did not seem to work any more. This failure further added to her depression, and she became obsessed with the idea that she had let her fiancé down by looking and behaving quite unlike her old self.

THE SYMPTOMS

Upon questioning Jane, other symptoms emerged. In spite of her extra 'padding' she could not seem to get warm. She found it difficult to get up in the morning, when she felt particularly tired and depressed with frequent headaches. Her friends and family had remarked how impatient and irritable she had become, and her memory and concentration were noticeably worsening. All these symptoms were new to Jane, having developed with the weight increase over the previous six to eight months.

THE TESTS

I requested a morning temperature check and a thyroid profile blood test. Jane's temperatures showed an average of 97.2°F (36.2°C) and her thyroid hormones were in the lower end of the normal range. Jane showed all the signs and symptoms of mild hypothyroidism.

THE TREATMENT

A nutritional programme was prescribed which included thyroid glandular supplements, and advice on regular exercise.

Within three months she was feeling more vital and less depressed. She had managed to lose 12lb on her usual diet.

By six months her blood thyroxine had improved by 25 per cent and her weight was down to 150lb. Jane was particularly encouraged that the diet was now working and she was hoping to regain a satisfactory weight before her wedding. Her mental lethargy and depression had slipped away and she was able to face the world upon waking with her old energy and enthusiasm.

Why are People Overweight?

Changes in weight which seem uncontrollable and inexplicable can be one of the most upsetting symptoms of an undiagnosed underactive thyroid. Many of us place a great deal of importance on our physical appearance; and even if your weight is not of great concern, you probably find it distressing to not be able to explain weight fluctuations.

There is a common stereotype that all those suffering from underactive thyroid are overweight – this is simply not true. If you are under the age of 40 you may in fact be underweight. Sometimes the metabolism is so sluggish that your use of dietary protein and other foods is inefficient and consequently you lose weight.

However, there is a tendency for the majority of middle-aged and elderly patients of both sexes with low grade hypothyroidism to put on unwanted weight. The thyroid does not directly cause obesity, but rather leads to symptoms such as tiredness, lack of energy and sugar cravings which in turn can lead you to become overweight.

Here are some further reasons why weight increase and thyroid are connected:

1   The metabolic sluggishness that results from hypothyroidism can cause digestive inefficiency and constipation.
2   The typical muscle and joint pain and stiffness tends to discourage the regular exercise that many patients rely on to control their weight.

3   The characteristic fatigue does not encourage activity. It is so
     easy 'not to bother' and all types of exercise and activity are
     usually reduced to a minimum.
4   If food is not converted to energy it is often converted into fat
     reserves. The poor gut absorption and candidiasis so common
     in hypothyroid, contributes to this conversion process.
5   Intestinal wind can increase the body size, and although the
     weight may not change – the appearance certainly can.
6   The efficient digestion of food requires the correct stomach
     acidity, pancreatic enzyme balance, gut absorption and bowel
     and bladder efficiency. These important areas of our
     metabolism can all be adversely affected by a depressed
     thyroid. The inevitable slowing of our metabolic rate leads to
     fluid retention, weight increase and a general reduction in our
     metabolic efficiency.
7   Depression is a common symptom of mild hypothyroidism,
     and depressed people usually have low self-confidence and
     suffer from anxiety. Unfortunately when these symptoms are
     experienced many of us turn to food for comfort, particular
     chocolate and sugar-rich foods. Alcohol is also taken for relief
     from anxiety. So a vicious circle can be established, involving
     the pattern opposite.
8   A decrease in brown fat. Brown fat consists of very specialized
     fat-burning tissue that is located around the neck, shoulders
     and upper spine, and around the vital organs including the
     kidney and heart. When the thyroid is underactive, the heat
     producing properties of this tissue tend to be reduced.

The Thyroid–Brain Link

We know that an underactive thyroid can contribute to weight
increase, depression and anxiety. The depression and mood changes
are in part caused by the resulting low levels of the neurotransmit-

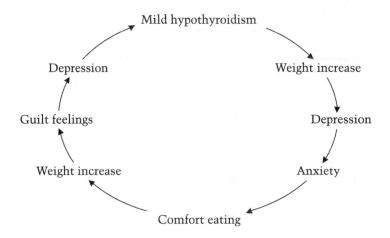

Figure 2: Hypothyroidism, weight gain and depression

ters in the brain. These include serotonin, GABA and noradrenaline. However, you may not realize that these neurotransmitters are also involved in appetite and taste regulation. For example, a decreased level of serotonin in the brain can cause a craving for sugar and car- bohydrates. This craving can lead to a pattern of eating that is so fre- quently – and mistakenly – attributed to low blood sugar.

How Many Calories Should I Consume?

Overweight patients frequently ask me for a calorie-controlled diet or a 'special foods' diet. Many are convinced that weight-loss would occur if they could only find and follow their 'ideal diet'. They believe that such a diet exists, and that the appropriate volume, vari- ety and combining of foods will solve their weight problem. This view has contributed to a vast array of diet books by celebrity authors, each of whom offers their own unique programme for weight loss. Unfortunately, effective and lasting weight loss depends on three elements. These being:

1 An efficient and healthy metabolism.
2 Regular activity and/or exercise.
3 A nutritionally balanced diet that is appropriate to our age, our lifestyle and our health history.

I find that many patients with mild hypothyroidism have great difficulty losing weight and perhaps more significantly, maintaining any new found slimness. Their metabolism can be so inefficient that I have known patients to increase weight even when following a low calorie diet plan consisting of no more than 800 calories daily.

Very low calorie diets tend to depress the metabolism and if the thyroid is already underactive, any weight loss on such a diet can only be very temporary. The weight loss–weight gain pattern so common to 'crash' dieting often tends to lower self-esteem, self-confidence and general vitality. The consequent frustration can lead to comfort eating and further depression, guilt and despair.

What Happens When you Diet?

Your body initially interprets dieting as a potential threat to its fuel supply. A need for emergency energy is therefore quickly recognized by the body. This energy is not obtained from fat, as the body is not able to rapidly utilize fat as energy. This role falls to a substance that is rarely discussed in diet books: **Glycogen or animal starch.** This is the chief carbohydrate reserve in humans, being stored primarily in liver and muscle tissue. Glycogen exists chiefly in solution with water, and our total reserves only amount to approximately 7–8lb. Although its energy value is less than half that of fat, glycogen converts to energy much more rapidly than fat. As a very small amount of energy is required to release water from the body's cells, dieting and the response to dieting leads to water loss and glycogen loss that is in solution in the water. This phenomena is well known to sportsmen, marathon runners can lose 10 or more pounds in one race. However, athletes prepare for such occurrences by following a very special pre-race diet for six or seven days. This involves a 'carbohydrate bleeding' phase for three days, which depletes the stores of glycogen by eating mainly protein-rich foods. This is then followed by three days of high carbohydrate eating, which serves to provide maximum starch reserves to be utilized during the race.

The rapid glycogen draining that occurs with many diets (particularly the low starch diets), coupled with the water loss, has two effects that can be very disturbing to the dieter:

1   A loss of glycogen can lower the body's blood sugar levels. This hypoglycaemia can cause fatigue, mood changes, dizziness and even faintness. Glucose is the main fuel for the nervous system. The brain, unlike our muscles, does not have a glucose reserve, so it is not surprising that many dieters experience depression, fatigue and mood changes.

2   Low levels of glycogen can trigger hunger pangs. Carbohydrate foods supply the glycogen stores and raise the blood sugar, providing us with a feeling of fullness and contentment. A high protein, low carbohydrate diet can cause a dieter to become ravenously hungry. Strict diets often lead to food craving.

Geoffrey Cannon has written:

In our minds we know the difference between going on a diet and being subjected to famine or starvation. But our bodies do not know the difference. When we go on a diet regime we activate the mechanisms in the body that protect us and preserves us in times of famine. And what does the body need to keep it going between times of famine? – Fat. The more often people diet, the more their bodies will protect the stores of fat.[1]

When discussing water loss in the context of dieting, it is worth noting that over 50 per cent of our weight consists of water.

Body fat contains very little water. For this reason women's bodies contain less water than men's. This is because the average woman has more body fat than the average man. Consequently an overweight person will hold less water than a lean person of similar weight. The proportion of water, fat and fat-free tissue lost with dieting varies from person to person according to their sex and the diet they followed.

Exercise and Dieting

Dieting can trigger your innate self-protection responses. Your body will adjust to deal with lifestyle changes, and what we do not use or need will take second place to the essential. An example being a sedentary, non-active person who does not use his/her muscles will tend to lose lean tissue (particularly muscle) when on a diet. This occurs simply because the dieter's body-wisdom does not recognize muscle tissue as being essential. Conversely an overweight individual's body will tend to preserve the fat it has become used to. If, however, the dieter is an active, sporting individual who makes use of his/her muscles, the muscle tissue will be seen by the metabolism as essential, and the lean muscle tissue loss will be minimal, but with more fat loss occurring.

The Thyroid and Weight Loss

I hope now it is becoming clear that the typical low carbohydrate, calorie-controlled diet is not ideal for you to lose weight.

Glycogen loss, temporary water loss and possible unwanted loss of lean muscle tissue can occur. The blood sugar can be reduced causing the many symptoms of hypoglycaemia that dieters can experience.

Essentially dieting slows the metabolism and mentally and physically we become more lethargic. This is our body's response to a reduced fuel supply.

To summarize, our metabolism can respond in six ways to a low calorie or low carbohydrate diet.

1   Glycogen loss occurs from muscle and liver tissue.
2   Water loss occurs.
3   Lean tissue (muscle) loss occurs.
4   Brown fat activity increases with complex carbohydrate food and decreases with high fat or protein foods.
5   The metabolism slows in response to the reduced fuel obtained from food.
6   Our metabolic rate, largely controlled by the thyroid, slows down through long-term dieting.

Many chronic dieters learn to recognize that their metabolism has adjusted to their dieting. Initial weight loss is usually followed by a period of static weight, even when the same reduced calorie or carbohydrate diet is being followed. Unfortunately the return to a 'normal' diet for non-active dieters, often leads to a rapid return to their original weight or even to a heavier weight. Although the dieting may have ended, their new reduced metabolic rate or tempo is still operating and

> using calories at a slower rate. The reduction in lean
> body mass as a result of the dieting causes a fall in the
> calories used for energy and a vicious circle is estab-
> lished.

You may be thinking: 'well yes, very interesting, but what about the thyroid?'. As discussed in other sections of this book, the thyroid is our metabolic clock. Therefore a metabolic slowing as a result of dieting can influence the thyroid. Conversely an existing under-active thyroid will lower metabolic activity, making dieting unsuc-cessful.

Brown Fat and the Thyroid

Research has been done over the last 20 years to show that when brown fat does not efficiently carry out its heat conversion role, the body's endocrine glands can be suspected. Underactivity of the adrenal glands and the thyroid gland being particularly implicated.

When this thyroid–brown fat link was identified, it was assumed that a person with inactive brown fat was also suffering with hypothyroidism and a prescription for thyroxine would solve the problem.

More recently, however, research has shown that the thyroid may be working normally, but the conversion of T_4 to T_3 may be ineffi-cient. This has lead to the view that re-balancing normal hormone conversion with the help of an optimum diet, supplement use and exercise, may be the answer, Jeffrey Bland believes that the minerals copper, zinc, iodine and selenium are of particular benefit.[2]

The amino acid tyrosine that combines with iodine to make T₃ and T₄ may also be responsible for increasing brown fat activity. It has been recommended for those individuals who show signs of low brown fat activity. As we know that this protein is so important for thyroid metabolism, it would appear to offer an invaluable dual role in treating obesity, particularly when the obesity is partly caused by underactivity of the thyroid gland.

Weight, Exercise and the Thyroid

Experiments involving low calorie diets have yielded significant information on the link between weight loss and the metabolic rate.

In 1919 F. G. Benedict placed 34 American student volunteers on a diet of 1,500 calories a day. After an average weight loss of 10 per cent (this took 60 days), their metabolic rate had fallen by 18 per cent[3]. More recently George K. Bray at UCLA put six very over-weight women on a 450 calorie diet for 24 days[4]. Their weight loss averaged seven per cent, but their metabolic output fell by 15 per cent. Such evidence confirms that dieting slows down our metabolic rate. In particular the vital organs are slowed, chiefly by a reduced use of oxygen. It follows that dieting cannot be seen as a healthy option. As the thyroid both regulates and reflects our metabolic rate, it is clear that a mildly underactive thyroid is incompatible with lasting weight reduction.

Weight loss should not depend on low calorie diets or low carbo-hydrate diets. Any attempts to lose weight should be directed towards normalizing the thyroid activity, eating a healthy balanced diet and following regular, preferably non-competitive, exercise. I have found that those patients who come to see me with a weight problem very often show low morning temperatures, and when they have in the past lost weight this was usually rapidly regained, sometimes with interest.

If you are a disillusioned dieter who has for some time yo-yoed from weight loss to weight gain on various diets, it is essential to ask yourself the following two simple questions in order to begin to assess whether you may be hypothyroid:

1 How much exercise do you do?
2 Are you cold or tired?

Now you have asked yourself these two questions you can begin to resolve your weight problem. Part Two shows you how to lose weight effectively *without disturbing your metabolism*, exercise efficiently, and begin to treat your mild hypothyroidism.

CHAPTER FOUR

'Why Do I Feel so Depressed?'

The Thyroid Gland and Your Emotions

Those of us who have never experienced the symptoms of clinical depression may liken depressive emotions to unhappiness. However, depression and unhappiness are completely different. This misunderstanding – or underestimation of the crippling effect of depression – can lead to a lack of sympathy with a depression victim. If you are depressed you might be told to 'take a holiday' or 'pull yourself together'. And if your depression persists – as it surely will without treatment – you may even be accused of self-centred sympathy seeking.

We all know about unhappiness. The causes are many and varied – we may have suffered a broken relationship, be frustrated in our career, or feel our life is unfulfilled – the list is endless. The common theme however, is that we usually know the cause of our unhappiness. Significantly the Shorter Oxford English Dictionary defines depression as 'A lowering in quality, vigour or amount: the state of being lowered'. Unhappiness is not mentioned. In fact many depressed patients are not always unhappy.

Those of you who may be suffering from clinical depression know that breaking the bonds of your depression cannot be achieved through a holiday or good night out with friends. If you suffer from depression *nothing and no-one* can make you feel better. This type of depression comes from within and cannot be solved by external factors. The medical term is 'clinical' or 'endogenous' depression. Depression which results from a external factor, such as divorce, bereavement or an known event is called 'secondary' or 'reactive' depression.

What Exactly is Depression?

Depression, like fatigue, is very difficult to define. We can only count on ourselves or loved ones to help us decide if we are indeed clinically depressed. Often the feeling of depression creeps onto us so slowly that we may not even be aware of what we used to feel like.

The American Psychiatric Association[1] lists eight typical symptoms associated with depression.These being:

1   Inappropriate weight gain or weight loss without obvious cause and with poor appetite.
2   Hyperactivity or hypoactivity.
3   Too little or too much sleep.
4   Reduced interest in normal activities including reduced libido.
5   Poor concentration.
6   Low self-esteem and feelings of inadequecy and guilt.
7   Suicidal tendencies and obsession with death.
8   Fatigue.

An individual suffering at least five of these symptoms for a minimum of four weeks could be diagnosed as a depressive. This criteria may seem rather vague and arbitrary, but it must be remembered that depression presents many symptoms that are difficult to categorize or measure.

Are you depressed?

A useful guideline for telling if you may be depressed is offered by Dr Ridha Arem in his book *The Thyroid Solution*[2].

Read through the following 22 questions and answer them as honestly and objectively as you can.

1 Are you tired all the time?
2 Have you lost interest or pleasure in activities that you used to enjoy?
3 Have you lost interest in sex?
4 Are you in a more or less constant sad mood?
5 Are you often irritable and become angry over trivial matters?
6 Do you experience crying spells?
7 Do you feel slowed down?
8 Do you have feelings of worthlessness?
9 Do you often experience a sense of guilt about things?
10 Has your appetite increased and/or have you gained weight?
11 Has your appetite decreased and/or have you lost weight?
12 Do you have difficulty with memory and/or difficulty concentrating on normal activities?
13 Do you have trouble making decisions, or do you feel inefficient?
14 Do you have trouble sleeping through the night?
15 Do you sleep too much (either going to bed too early or sleeping too late)?
16 Do you wish you were dead?
17 Do you think about harming or killing yourself?
18 Do you feel like a failure?
19 Do you feel pessimistic or hopeless most of the time?
20 Are you too critical of yourself, or do you dislike yourself?
21 Do you feel that you are being punished?
22 Have you become very sensitive to criticism or rejection?

If you answered 'yes' to five or more of the above questions you may be depressed. It would be wise to talk to a health professional or doctor about these feelings.

This list is very helpful to assess your symptoms as an aid to diagnosis. However, to make the process easier I believe that there are six key symptoms that are common to those who are depressed. These being:

1   Low libido
2   Poor concentration and memory
3   Mental and physical fatigue
4   Moodiness and low self-esteem
5   Unexpected weight gain or weight loss
6   Disturbances of the metabolism, including appetite, sleep patterns, bowels and immune efficiency.

Depression and Fatigue

I have never seen a patient with clinical or endogenous depression who was full of vitality. Depressed people are tired people. They are also usually anxious and perplexed people. This anxiety stems partly from a failure to identify the cause of their depression, a frequent comment being 'I have no reason to be depressed'. Often their work, family, and lifestyle provide all they would wish for.

Depression – Mind or Body?

The symptoms of clinical depression may be well defined and recognized, but the causes of depression are the subject of controversy within the medical profession and the complementary professions.

The central point of debate that has split doctors, psychiatrists and the many other therapists who treat depression into two opposing groups, is simply the question of mind versus body.

The key issue that fuels the controversy involves the following question:

With depression does the mind affect the body or does the body affect the mind?

Many doctors believe that depression is a personality disorder and the accompanying physical symptoms that are manifested can be effectively treated with antidepressant drugs. As a result of this reasoning, I quite often see patients who have been prescribed Amitriptyline or Prozac for backache and bowel disorders.

This view is supported by the fact that many patients experience symptom-relief from their physical symptoms when taking antidepressants. Clinical trials have confirmed that irritable bowel syndrome (IBS) and Crohn's disease, which have long thought to be stress induced, can be improved under hypnotherapy.

However, there is overwhelming evidence to support the view that it is the body that influences the mind.

It should be realized that every thought and emotion we experience is preceded by a chemical change in the brain cells. As with all the other organs in the body, the brain only functions normally when the optimum fuel is available. We all recognize and accept that inappropriate abnormalities in our blood chemistry can alter our personality. This can be seen in alcoholism and low blood sugar as well as with the side effects of drugs and hormonal imbalances (e.g. PMS). These changes are usually transient, but the many substances that can cause depression can lead to long-term symptoms.

Depression occurs chiefly as a result of physiological, not psychological, malfunction. In common with many health problems that previously carried a psychiatric 'label' (such as autism, schizophrenia, attention deficit disorder and hyperactivity), depression is now seen as a nutritional or biochemical disorder.

What Happens When I Get Depressed?

The brain relays electrical messages from one nerve cell to the next with the aid of neurotransmitters. There exist around 40 of these substances whose role is to cover the space between the nerves (the synapses) so that the signals pass unimpeded.

Depression is thought by many doctors, nutritionists and researchers to be caused by a deficiency of neurotransmitters. Up until quite recently it was assumed that these vital substances occur in the brain and are not dependent on, or directly influenced by, the food we eat. The blood–brain barrier was always thought to insulate the brain from the effects of incorrect diet. We now know that neurotransmitters can be deficient, and that they can be influenced by nutritional supplements and dietary manipulation.

Examples of neurotransmitters include serotonin, dopamine, acetycholine, epinephine (adrenaline), glycine and GABA (gamma-aminobutyric acid) and the endorphins. Prescription drugs for depression influence these important chemicals.

ANTIDEPRESSANT DRUGS
The antidepressant drugs in common use fall into three separate drug groups. Each group has a different mode of action on the brain chemistry.

1 MONOAMINE OXIDASE (MAO) INHIBITORS
These drugs inhibit the enzyme (MAO), that is responsible for the metabolic breakdown of the neurotransmitters, including serotonin, dopamine, epinephrine (adrenalin) and

norepinephrine (noradrenaline). This allows for more of the neurotransmitters to be in circulation. The best known drugs in this group are Parnate, Nardil and Parstelin.

2   TRICYCLICS
    This group of drugs leads to reduction of histamine and an increase in noradrenaline. The most common of these drugs include Amitriptyline, Imipramine and Anafranil.

3   SELECTIVE SEROTONIN RE-UPTAKE INHIBITORS (SSRI's)
    These work by selectively reducing the uptake of Serotonin, thus allowing more Serotonin into the circulation. The best known drug in this group is Prozac.

The Thyroid and Depression

If you suffer from low grade hypothyroidism your entire body can feel mentally and physically depressed. In fact, hypothyroidism depresses the whole metabolism. As I have mentioned (see page 10) hypothyroidism can mean that T_3 is not converted efficiently from T_4 at cell level. T_3 (Triiodthyronine) is a powerful hormone in the body and therefore one key to understanding depression.

The T_3 hormone is itself a neurotransmitter as potent in its action as serotonin. However, it is also essential to maintain the levels of serotonin and noradrenaline in the brain. If you do not have enough T_3 you will be lacking in these two hormones. Noradrenaline deficiency is seen as a major cause of depression. Therefore it is vital to ascertain whether you may have low grade hypothyroidism in order to effectively treat depression.

PETER'S STORY

Peter was an international sales manager for a computer hardware company. His work was very tiring and very stressful. He had targets to set, problems to solve and planes to catch on a daily basis. Aged 50 and at the top of his promotion curve, there were several younger colleagues eager to succeed him. Being unmarried and well paid he tended to rely on restaurant meals, usually taken as working lunches and dinners. In common with many business executives he had settled into a habit of eating rich food with wine and he supported his flagging nervous system with 10–12 sweet coffees and 25–30 cigarettes daily. Not surprisingly he had been overweight for 20 years. However, his weight was not his chief concern. For the previous two years he had suffered stomach pain, heartburn, fullness after meals, fatigue, complete loss of libido, and neck and shoulder stiffness and pain.

A combination of symptoms and work pressures had contributed to his ever-worsening depression. He explained that his chief concern was whether the depression was a cause or a symptom of his ill health.

When I examined Peter he weighed 210lb. His height was six foot with medium-sized hands and feet, so I estimated that he was 35lb overweight. His blood pressure was too high at 180 over 95 and he looked and sounded tired and depressed.

Although he did not complain of feeling unduly cold, I requested his morning temperatures. I also requested a full blood screen including haematology (to assess anaemia), a mineral/vitamin profile, and a biochemistry and thyroid profile. Also a heliobactor pylori antibody test to check for stomach ulcers.

He was requested to attend a specialist diagnostic unit in London to have a gastric function test that measured stomach acidity, pancreatic enzyme activity and stomach emptying speed.

Peter had consulted his own doctor and a gastroscopy had been requested. No stomach ulceration was present. He was given a diagnosis of stress gastritis with reflux, and treated with antacids.

The past history had included a bout of glandular fever 10 years earlier, and a brief course of antidepressants three years earlier.

Peter's test results showed that he had several problems in need of attention. The thyroid hormone T₄ was right at the bottom of the range, and his average morning temperature was 97.2°F (36.2°C) The blood lipids were all raised, these included the total cholesterol and the bad LDL fraction, also the triglycerides. His haemoglobin was low, confirming borderline anaemia.

The gastric function test showed a high stomach acid level (low pH) and a pancreatic enzyme deficiency. The stomach emptying speed was normal and fortunately the heliobactor test was negative.

I prescribed a full nutritional programme for Peter which included the following:

* Advice on better eating, a low fat and low sugar diet similar to the food combining pattern.
* Strict avoidance of caffeine, tobacco and alcohol.
* Avoiding business discussions when eating.
* Supplementary iron, multi-vitamins and minerals, thyroid and adrenal glandulars and omega 3 (fish oils) for blood fat control.
* A two phase digestive enzyme formula was recommended.

A substance in cigarette smoke known as thyocyamide can inhibit the thyroid gland. Smoking also destroys vitamin C at the rate of 25mg per cigarette.

Stress can exhaust the adrenals and cause hypoglycaemia with subsequent potassium loss and sodium retention. This process leads to fluid retention, excess weight and raised blood pressure. High cholesterol and triglycerides can cause a narrowing of blood vessels and raised blood pressure.

The exact cause of Peter's symptoms was unclear. The suspected post-viral fatigue following glandular fever, together with his poor digestion and anaemia, may have depressed his metabolic rate and predisposed him to mild hypothyroidism. He had subsequently developed a vicious circle of fatigue, stress, incorrect eating and more fatigue, coupled with depression. The priority was to improve his vitality to enable him to do his work without undue effort or stress.

Although his neck and shoulder pain was partly caused by his thyroid, Peter was also unfit as a result of lack of exercise. I therefore arranged a course of massage and advised him to make use of the swimming facilities offered at the various hotels that he used.

Within four months Peter had lost 20lb, and tests confirmed that he was progressing well. He felt more vital and optimistic and seemed to be enjoying his new healthier lifestyle. As the causes of his depression slipped away so his mood improved.

Nutrition, Lifestyle and Depression

There are many nutritional, environmental and metabolic factors which can contribute to depression by influencing the availability of neurotransmitters. Nearly everything we consume has the capability to affect our neurotransmitters. Although it is not possible to assess every factor, research has shown that vitamins, minerals, amino acids, caffeine, tobacco and alchohol can all have a significant effect on our state of mind.

Vitamins, Minerals and Amino Acids

VITAMIN B1 (THIAMINE)
Depression is common in thiamine deficiency, particularly depression of the elderly. In common with other 'B' vitamins, thiamine may show normal levels in the blood but inappropriately low levels in the central nervous system and other tissue. The blood is given priority by the body's systems and as a result blood tests and 'normal ranges' can be misleading.

VITAMIN B₂ (RIBOFLAVIN)

Also linked to depression, and often found to be deficient in mental patients.

VITAMIN B₃ (NIACIN)

Niacin deficiency causes decreased metabolic energy in the b
rain. Supplementing this vitamin increases the tryptophan status as niacin is synthesized for the production of the neurotransmitter serotonin. Deficiency of B₃ can *also* contribute to memory loss and anxiety.

VITAMIN B₅ (PANTOTHENIC ACID)

Another 'B' vitamin that contributes to depression when deficient.

VITAMIN B₆ (PYRIDOXINE)

Psychiatric patients with vitamin B₆ deficiency suffer from endogenous depression. This vitamin is prescribed to treat depression caused by the birthpill as the pill can cause tryptophan destruction.

> Tryptophan is an amino acid (a protein building block), and it is one of the metabolic precursors for serotonin.

BIOTIN

Deficiency can cause depression and extreme fatigue, with a great desire to sleep.

FOLIC ACID

Folic acid is the commonest nutrient deficiency in the world. Studies have shown up to 30 per cent of psychiatric patients to be deficient in this vitamin. Deficiency is known to lower the neurotransmitter serotonin and can cause symptoms of depression, poor memory, dementia and insomnia.

VITAMIN B₁₂

Vitamin B₁₂ is another common vitamin deficiency, particularly amongst the elderly, and even mild non anaemic levels may cause depression. Other symptoms can include fatigue, confusion, memory loss and delusions. Severe deficiency is termed 'pernicious anaemia'.

VITAMIN C

One of the earliest symptoms to show in scurvy (vitamin C deficiency) is depression. Mild scurvy is not uncommon, particularly amongst the elderly. Trials have confirmed that supplementary vitamin C can ease the symptoms of depression.

Mineral Deficiency

Deficiency of the minerals calcium, magnesium, potassium and iron have all been linked with depression. High levels of magnesium, vanadium, mercury, lead and cadmium are also known to cause depression.

Iron Deficient Anaemia

Iron deficient anaemia is the commonest anaemia causing mental and physical fatigue. Patients with anaemia can also become depressed. The mechanism for this is not fully understood, however, it is known that even after the blood is normalized the depression can persist for many months.

Amino Acids

The amino acids are building blocks or fractions that make up protein. There are over 100 amino acids but 20 are needed before the body can synthesize protein.

The nine 'essential' amino acids cannot be synthesized by adults and can only be obtained through the diet. These include isoleucine,

leucine, lysine, methionine, phenylalanine (DLPA), threonine, tryptophan and valine.

Each amino acid has its own unique function and activities within the body. They also offer predictable therapeutic effects. The availability of the essential amino acids depends on an optimum diet. Low protein diets can contribute to clinical depression.

> Great care should be taken when supplementing with amino acids. They can adversely interact with antidepressant drugs and certain foods. They can be more effective when taken alongside specific co-factors e.g. vitamins. The timing of the dose, and need to avoid mixing certain amino acids, can be important.

Amino acids of special value in the treatment of depression include tryptophan, tyrosine, glutamine, phenylalanine and methionine. Phenylalanine can convert into phenylethylamine or PEA. This compound can raise the libido and acts as a natural antidepressant. Low levels have been identified in depressed patients. Chocolate contains PEA which may perhaps explain chocolate's mild aphrodisiac properties and romantic overtones. Proline is also recommended for short-term depression. Low taurine levels have been found in depressed patients and the amino acid carnitine has been recommended for use in hypothyroid depression.

The amino acids are the precursors or building blocks of many of the brain's neurotransmitters, and although further research is needed, they may in the future provide effective drug-free treatment for clinical depression.

Caffeine

Many studies have linked caffeine consumption to depression and other mental and emotional symptoms. It has been demonstrated that consuming six cups of coffee or 10 cups of tea (600–700mg of caffeine) daily may lead to depression.

> The use of free coffee dispensing machines in offices and factories provides a tempting source of caffeine-rich drinks. I have spoken to patients who regularly drink 20 to 30 cups of coffee each day. Caffeine raises blood sugar, reduces the appetite for food and can contribute to adrenal exhaustion and subsequent low blood sugar (hypoglycaemia).

Cola drinks also contain caffeine, usually around 35mg to 40mg per glass. A high intake of caffeine can lead to a condition known as 'caffeinism'. This term describes a group of symptoms similar to adrenal exhaustion (see page 209) and 'burnt-out' syndrome. The symptoms can include the following:

* Anxiety and panic feelings
* Hyperventilation
* Headaches
* Nervous tics and twitches
* Rapid heart beat
* Depression or general irritability
* Nocturnal 'restless leg syndrome'

Tobacco

A great deal has been written about the dangers of smoking. Not surprisingly, the main topic has been cancer and the effects of nicotine on lung health. There are, however, other side effects resulting from smoking and in the context of mood and depression, smoking can play a significant role.

The nicotine from one cigarette can cause an increase in the blood sugar (due to stimulation of the adrenal glands). A surge of 36 per cent to 75 per cent for up to 20 minutes has been demonstrated in controlled studies. The type of surge triggered by smoking is usually followed by a subsequent fall in the blood sugar level. This can lead to a see-saw effect. The smoker has a cigarette, obtains a quick 'lift' but after 15–20 minutes feels the urge for another lift. Unfortunately the inbetween falls in the blood sugar create a desire for anything that will quickly raise the levels again. This includes caffeine, sugar, chocolate and alcohol. Statistics show that smokers drink twice the amount of coffee and alcohol than non-smokers.

Smoking also causes vitamin C loss. This has been identified as 25mg of vitamin C per cigarette. The role of vitamin C deficiency in depression is discussed on page 52.

Leon Chaitow defines the results of smoking as 'a vast number of interlocking hormonal and biochemical changes[3]'.

This sentence describes perfectly the complexity of imbalances caused by smoking, and features depression as one of the commonest symptoms.

Alcohol

There is no doubt that alcohol significantly influences our mood, we have all experienced (or seen other people experience) the effects of excessive alcohol consumption. Poor co-ordination, fatigue, mood changes and slurred speech are typical symptoms. Excessive alcohol can also cause low blood sugar. Similar to caffeine consumption, the rebound fall in the blood sugar creates a craving for sugar-rich foods or drinks. The alcoholic can thus experience many symptoms, including depression. This is particularly evident when withdrawing from alcohol, or when the blood sugar falls to a low level after sleep, better known as the familiar 'hangover'.

Food Intolerances

Research studies have shown that up to 30 per cent of depressed patients suffer from food intolerances or sensitivities.

As is so often the case with the many symptoms associated with food intolerances, no specific food has been implicated in causing depression. Exactly how or why food influences our mental health is seen as a complex and controversial topic. However, it is generally recognized that food intolerances can cause depression, anxiety, hyperactivity in children, confusion and mood swings.

The exact causal link between food intolerance and mental health has yet to be established, however, depression and other symptoms have been predictably induced with food avoidance-provocation procedures. Although many researchers and clinicians believe food intolerances are 'all in the mind', the following list outlines some of the ways that our food can adversely affect mental health, including depression.

1 Low stomach acid (achlorhydria). Inadequate stomach acid can lead to the development of new food intolerances. This can be caused by incomplete protein digestion.
2 Caffeinism (see page 54).
3 Allergy or reaction to food additives e.g. azo dyes, monosodium glutamate and aspartame.
4 Low blood sugar (hypoglycaemia).
5 Specific reaction to substances in food known as vasoactive (affecting blood vessels) amines (e.g. histamine). Significantly, the tricyclic antidepressant drugs are powerful antihistamines.

6   Leaky gut (increased intestinal permeability) or malabsorption (toxic gut), leading to the abnormal absorption of nutrients.

Sugar

Excessive sugar consumption can cause low blood sugar, a common cause of depression and many other symptoms. Studies have shown that significant mood change can develop as a result of taking excessive sugar. Conversely depression can improve with a sugar free diet.

Fat

Trials have shown that depression can be improved by taking evening primrose oil (a source of omega-6 fatty acid). The high animal fat and refined starch content of the western diet has been linked to the increasing figures for depressive illness. This may in part be caused by a reduction in the omega-3 fatty acids (fish oils) characteristic of such a diet. We hear a great deal of comment on the dangers of elevated blood cholesterol. An Italian study has demonstrated, however, that many potential suicide victims had a very low serum cholesterol.

It has been demonstrated that those who follow a very low fat diet run the risk of losing their ability to absorb the neurotransmitter serotonin.

If you feel that your diet and lifestyle may be contributing to your mood, please turn to chapter ten on recovery through diet.

Hormones and Depression

Imbalance of hormones in the body can cause depression.

The Adrenal Glands

DHEA (dehydroepiandrosterone) is the most prevalent adrenal hormone, with small amounts being produced by the ovaries. It acts as a precursor steroid or 'buffer' hormone and interacts with other hormones. It can be converted by the body into oestrogen, progesterone, testosterone (the sex hormone) and cortisone. The levels of DHEA in the body fall as we age.

Clinical research has suggested that it may be of value in treating fatigue, depression, poor concentration and memory and mood changes. It is also being considered for the treatment of psoriasis, high blood pressure, obesity, diabetes, multiple sclerosis, Alzheimer's disease and in lowering blood cholesterol.

Some American physicians claim that at least 50 per cent of their depressed patients are low in DHEA.

ADRENALINE (EPINEPHRINE)

This hormone has two major roles. It is released in response to hypoglycaemia, stress and other stimuli (the body's 'flight and fight' response). It also serves as a neurotransmitter (classed as a catecholamine) being released into the central nervous system to facilitate nerve transmittion. Hypoadrenalism can contribute to poor stress handling, hypoglycaemia, anxiety and depression.

NORADRENALINE (NOREPINEPHRINE)

Another adrenal hormone, released by the brain neurones and the adrenal gland. It is also a neurotransmitter (and classed as a catecholamine). The thyroid gland controls the levels of noradrenaline. Deficiency of this hormone is seen by many doctors as a major cause of depression.

CORTISOL

This major adrenal hormone that can be synthesized to cortisone is involved in the metabolism of fats, carbohydrates and proteins. (When used as a drug it is referred to as hydrocortisone.)

High levels of cortisol cause similar symptoms to those caused by taking excessive cortisone as a drug. These include general nervousness, insomnia and depression.

PREGNENOLONE

In common with DHEA, oestrogen and testosterone, pregnenolone is synthesized from cholesterol. Seen as the 'mother' hormone, this important steroid is prescribed for any illness or symptom for which cortisone is prescribed. These include asthma, arthritis, depression, fatigue, SLE (Lupus) and many others. Although not so speedy in its effect or so powerful as cortisone, it does not produce the side effects that are characteristic of cortisone therapy. These can include high blood pressure, fluid retention, weight increase, immune breakdown and blood vessel brittleness, loss of bone mass and a tendency to diabetes. Pregnenolone was initially researched in the 1940s as a treatment for arthritis. However, as a natural substance it could not be patented, and cortisone (prednisolone) soon replaced it as the treatment of choice.

The Oral Contraceptive-Birth Pill

The birth pill causes three main groups of side effects that can contribute to depression, these being:

1   Long-term use of the birth pill can cause numerous nutrient imbalances, notably deficiencies of Vitamin B_2, B_6, Folic Acid and B_{12}, vitamin C and iron. Vitamin A and copper can be increased with its use.

2   Oestrogen is known to influence blood sugar metabolism, playing a role in hypoglycaemia, which contributes to depression.

3   Vitamin B$_6$ status can be disturbed by the birth-control pill and tryptophan can be destroyed. For this reason, vitamin B$_6$ is prescribed to reduce the side effects of the birth-control pill.

Other Causes of Depression

Biochemical imbalances in our environment can lead to the nutrient deficiencies that cause depression. Drug side effects, chemical pollutants, food additives, soil depletion and toxic metals in our environment all serve to threaten our biochemistry leading to the deficiencies discussed earlier in this chapter.

CHAPTER FIVE

'Why do I Never Feel Like Sex Anymore?'

The Thyroid Gland and Your Sex Drive

If you suffer from an underactive thyroid nearly every aspect of your body will be altered – this includes your sex drive. When your body is not working properly, the natural desire to reproduce is one of the first aspects of your health to suffer. This loss of libido can cause great distress and worry, especially when you do not understand the cause. The thyroid influences your sex drive on three levels:

1   Direct changes to brain chemistry.
2   Changes to the levels of the sex hormones.
3   Indirect effects as a result of general hypothyroid symptoms.

Let us look at each of these levels in turn.

Direct Changes to Brain Chemistry

Virtually any sexual trigger, whether a caress, a scent or simply a thought has the potential to cause the release of brain transmitters that stimulate the autonomic nervous system.

> The autonomic nervous system consists of a self-sufficient system that functions independently from the rest of our nervous system. One of its functions is to control of the endocrine (hormonal) system.

When this occurs we can experience a wide variety of responses that we would call sexual stimulation. These include an increase in our breathing and heart rate, heightened skin sensitivity, lubrication of the woman's genitalia and an increased flow of blood to the penis causing an erection.

All these responses depend on optimum levels of the thyroid hormones. When the thyroid becomes underactive, the sexual signals do not trigger the autonomic response, and the sexual urge and satisfaction is diminished or ceases altogether. This reduction in sex drive is not only apparent on a physical level (i.e. intercourse), but can lead to a general decline in sexual excitement, healthy sexual fantasising, and sexual satisfaction.

The Sex Hormones

These include oestrogen, progesterone and testosterone. All these hormones – plus the adrenal hormone DHEA – are made from cholesterol.

> Although progesterone is a single hormone, the word oestrogen describes a whole family of around 20 hormones. These are all different in chemical structure and function. Examples are oestriol, oestradial and oestrone.

Deficiencies of all or any one of these hormones, can occur with hypothyroidism. Oestrogen and testosterone play important roles in the development of male and female sexual characteristics.

Men require more testosterone than oestrogen and for women the opposite applies.

> There exists a delicate balance between the two hormones in both sexes. It has been postulated that the current decreasing levels in the male sperm count and male testosterone in 'civilized' nations can be explained by the increasing presence of foreign oestrogen-like substances in our environment. These are known as 'xenoestrogens' which contain an extremely poisonous compound known as phenol. This substance can be found in dyes, disinfectants, plastics, agricultural pesticides, petrochemical pollutants and certain drugs.

Progesterone

Progesterone (and oestrogen) are mainly produced in the ovaries. Small amounts are also released from the adrenal glands.

> The adrenal supply of oestrogen assumes a special importance when during menopause the ovaries virtually cease to function.

The role of the two hormones is key in our understanding of a woman's menstrual cycle. Oestrogen dominates the initial two weeks and progesterone is the dominant hormone for the final two weeks of the month.

Dr John R. Lee – who is known for his work on oestrogen dominance – has stated that a low progesterone level is often misdiagnosed as thyroid deficiency[1]. Progesterone is responsible for the female sex drive, not oestrogen as is commonly assumed.

The thyroid hormones and progesterone complement each other. Conversely oestrogen production can be stimulated by a thyroid deficiency. Any excess of oestrogen, referred to as 'oestrogen dominance', further lowers available progesterone levels. This unopposed oestrogen is normally balanced by progesterone but when the balance fails the following symptoms can develop:

1   Weight increase
2   Thyroid depression
3   Fluid retention
4   Joint and muscle pain
5   Poor circulation
6   Reduced sex drive
7   Headaches
8   Depression
9   Low blood sugar
10   Potassium–sodium imbalance
11   Zinc and copper reductions

Significantly the body can convert progesterone into oestrogen. For this and other reasons many American doctors are questioning the need for oestrogen supplementation. Many 'good' and safe oestrogens are available through our food. These phytoestrogens are chiefly found in soya, which may explain the low levels of menstrual and menopausal symptoms experienced by Japanese women; soya products tend to dominate Japanese cuisine. These good oestrogens are not carcinogenic, in fact they can provide a protective influence against female cancers.

Testosterone

This essentially male hormone can be decreased with hypothyroidism resulting in a reduced sexual potency in men in addition to many other symptoms.

Summary

1   The thyroid can depress the levels of all the sex hormones.
2   The symptoms of oestrogen dominance and/or reduced progesterone are similar to, and often mistaken for, hypothyroidism.
3   Supplementary progesterone (as an ointment) can be a safe and effective method of restoring any imbalance between oestrogen and progesterone.
4   The role of the thyroid hormones on brain function, the autonomic nervous system and on the male and female sex hormones explains many of the sexual symptoms that can occur with hypothyroidism.

Indirect Effects

Aside from the more specific hormonal influences resulting from hypothyroidism, there exists a host of general thyroid symptoms that can indirectly reduce sexual desire and potency in both sexes.

Fatigue, as we know, is the commonest symptom of hypothyroidism. Exhaustion and sex do not go well together. A partner's refusal as a result of fatigue, can reduce self-esteem, increase feelings of rejection, and cause resentment and frustration. If this scenario occurs occasionally it may not be significant, but the chronic fatigue resulting from an underactive thyroid is constant and unrelenting.

How we look is also an important component in sexual desire and activity. Many hypothyroid patients are embarrassed by their appearance, they may be overweight with dry skin and lifeless hair.

Vaginal lubrication depends on efficient functioning of the thyroid hormones, if this is diminished, vaginal dryness with painful intercourse may result. If intercourse ceases to be enjoyable, anxiety and guilt can result from an increasingly one-sided partnership.

Depression reduces the desire for sex. It can become increasingly difficult to maintain a satisfactory, loving relationship when one's partner is depressed as a result of an underactive thyroid.

There are other routes for hypothyroidism to influence male and female sexuality. Reduced blood flow to the pelvis can adversely affect sex, and blood vessel narrowing (atherosclerosis) that can be linked to thyroid function can be the cause.

Hypothyroidism can cause high blood pressure and some of the drugs prescribed for raised blood pressure can reduce the libido.

Stress has been shown to reduce the thyroid hormones and the subsequent sex drive. The body coldness and the frequent headaches that accompany hypothyroid can further reduce sexual desire and performance. It is therefore not too surprising that thyroid problems can diminish sexual desire and satisfaction.

CLARE'S STORY

Clare looked older than her years. Although she was just 30 years old when she first consulted me, she looked nearer 40. She was obviously underweight with a lined, gaunt face and a postural slump to her shoulders that said 'I can't be bothered'.

She complained of fatigue, pain and stiffness in the elbows and knees and a frequent 'shaky' and anxious feeling with missing meals, and often before meals. She always felt cold, and suffered occasional panic attacks. Her concentration was poor, and as her work involved working with computers she felt that she may have to seek easier, lower paid employment. However, her main concern was her marriage. She had been married for 18 months and within two or three months after the marriage her weight loss and other symptoms developed.

Clare's husband who was 10 years older than Clare, was not considered 'suitable' by her family. This attitude contributed to the stress that Clare had experienced since her marriage, and made worse as her husband had reacted to the rejection by refusing to meet her parents. Clare loved her parents and she loved her husband, so she felt desperately unhappy at a situation that she considered was her fault.

EXAMINATION

Although Clare's height was five foot five inches, she only weighed 94lb. Her blood pressure at the consultation was low being 100 over 75. Her weight when she married had been 118lb. So in the space of eighteen months Clare had lost 24lb.

She had always enjoyed good health up to her marriage, so it seemed likely that the stress she had suffered was a possible cause of her present symptoms. Unfortunately her family conflicts were not her only cause of stress. Over the previous year she had lost any interest in the sexual side of her marriage, and although she loved her husband, she did not welcome sexual contact with him.

DIET

Clare hated cooking. She had lived with her parents before her marriage and enjoyed an excellent diet. Now her diet was poor, consisting of coffee for breakfast, crisps, biscuits and coffee for lunch and a dinner that usually consisted of poor quality convenience food. With access to a free coffee dispenser in her office she consumed 15 to 20 coffees daily with added sugar, and she satisfied her chocolate craving with two to three chocolate bars each day. Fortunately she did not smoke. However, she drank approximately 30 units of red wine each week.

DIAGNOSIS

Clare presented a common dual problem, mild hypothyroidism coupled with adrenal exhaustion and resulting low blood sugar. The chronic stress had depleted her adrenal efficiency and her high sugar diet was causing swings in her blood sugar that were out of control. Her metabolism was not able to control the sugar surges and the subsequent reactive falls in the blood sugar served to increase her sugar craving. A vicious circle had been established and she turned to sugar and caffeine in place of regular meals for a rapid energy supply.

The thyroid had been pulled into this imbalance. Her metabolism, weight and vitality had all diminished, and her thyroid matched this by slowing down. This was confirmed in a blood thyroid profile. Clare's results were at the bottom of the normal range and her average morning temperature was also too low.

TREATMENT

Clare was prescribed thyroid and adrenal glandular capsules and a GTF Complex (glucose tolerance factor, see page 225). She was urged to change her diet in favour of regular low sugar meals, and to avoid coffee and sugar. The chocolates had to go, and her alcohol was reduced to one glass of red wine with her dinner.

Our metabolism regards the sex drive as a luxury function, and therefore non-essential. In Clare's exhausted stressed state, her sexual urge and interest had fallen to zero. The underactive thyroid also played a part in suppressing her libido.

Clare and her husband sought marriage counselling and over a period of three months Clare began to increase her weight and vitality. Her husband was delighted with the changes and their obvious happiness encouraged her parents to alter their attitude towards him.

Clare's case demonstrates how easily the mind–body balance can be disturbed. I have seen patients undergo a personality improvement simply with an improved diet. The thyroid effect on symptoms is a two-way influence. Stress, illness and poor nutrition can all slow the thyroid. This can depress the adrenal hormones and the sex hormones. When such a vicious circle is established, the symptoms can reflect a disturbed mind as much as a disturbed body.

The Thyroid Gland,
Menstrual Patterns and PMS

Menstrual Symptoms

Low grade hypothyroidism can lead to a diversity of unpleasant menstrual symptoms which can cause women considerable pain and unhappiness. If you are a woman and suffer from heavy or extended periods, menstrual cramps, irregular cycles or painful periods, then you may benefit from thyroid therapy.

The connection between menstrual symptoms and hypothyroidism was established and treated as early as the 1880s. A report published by the Clinical Society of London in 1888 showed a 35 per cent incidence of menstrual symptoms in women with hypothyroidism. Work from Broda Barnes demonstrated the relief many women receive through thyroid treatment. He also showed that women who discontinued thyroid treatment often suffered a reoccurrence of their menstrual symptoms. Please see page 74 for more details of this and other historical research.

There is also some evidence to show that hypothyroidism contributes to PMS, and for some women may even be the main cause of this common condition.

What is PMS?

No precise definition exists for PMS although in excess of 100 symptoms have been attributed to the problem, and a variety of factors have been suggested as possible causes.

The pituitary gland is the common master gland for both the thyroid and the ovaries, it is therefore not surprising that an underactive thyroid can play a part in PMS. When looking at the symptoms and the symptom categories that are characteristic of PMS you will not fail to notice the similarities to the symptoms of hypothyroidism. Significantly, as you will read, PMS is thought by many doctors to be caused by a low progesterone deficiency yet low progesterone is frequently misdiagnosed as hypothyroidism.

PMS Symptoms

More than 100 symptoms have been identified and there is no need to list them all. However, Dr Guy Abraham has identified four subgroups or categories of PMS symptoms[2]. These he defined in the table below, the title of each group being determined by the chief symptom.

Common symptoms of PMS

1. PMS (Anxiety)
Symptoms include:
Mood swings, anxiety, headaches, insomnia and general nervous tension.

2. PMS (Depression)
Symptoms include:
Depression, poor memory and general sense of confusion and low self-esteem.

3. PMS (Craving)

Symptoms include:

Craving for sugar and chocolate, headaches, fatigue, dizziness, palpitations and an increased appetite

4. PMS Excessive body water content (hyperhydration)

Symptoms include:

Weight increase, extremity swelling, stomach bloating and breast tenderness.

You may now be thinking, 'Where does the thyroid feature in these groups?' This will become clear when the background characteristics of the four groups are outlined. Compare this table with the one below.

Causes of PMS symptoms

1. PMS (Anxiety)

Usually elevated oestrogen and reduced progesterone.

2. PMS (Depression)

Can be associated with low thyroid hormones. Also lead toxicity is sometimes found.

3. PMS (Craving)

Associated with a tendency toward low blood sugar, and low levels of magnesium and sometimes chromium.

4. PMS (Hyperhydration)

Associated with raised blood aldosterone.

A raised sodium and a low potassium with a tendency towards fluid retention.

> Aldosterone is a steroid hormone produced by the adrenal glands. Its role is to assist the regulation of the sodium-potassium balance in the blood. If the balance is lost we either lose fluid and need sodium (salt, as in hot climates), or retain water and need potassium.

Although the thyroid's influence is only directly involved in the PMS Depression group, there is also an indirect association with the PMS Anxiety group and with the PMS Craving group.

Treatment

Many nutritional treatment strategies have been suggested for the treatment of PMS. These include low sugar diets, the avoidance of animal fat, and the taking of omega-6 fatty acids, vitamins, minerals and natural diuretics (to reduce fluid).

However, I would recommend that when looking to diagnose and treat chronic PMS, a good starting point is to ask your doctor or complementary health practitioner to assess your thyroid function though the means of a blood test, and a morning temperature check (see chapter nine).

Although thyroid underactivity is rarely the sole cause of PMS, if you do suffer from any reduction in thyroid efficiency your PMS symptoms will, as a result, be made worse. The identification and treatment of low grade hypothyroidism is an essential first step in treating your PMS.

HISTORICAL EVIDENCE

As mentioned, the connection between menstrual symptoms and hypothyroidism was established and treated from the 1880s. The Clinical Society of London in 1888 investigating 'myxoedema' published a report showing a 35 per cent incidence of menstrual symptoms in women with hypothyroidism. In 1927 a report by Gardiner Hill and Smith showed an incidence of 78 per cent with heavy periods in hypothyroid patients[3].

Broda Barnes in a report published in 1949 showed that a diversity of menstrual symptoms including menstrual cramps, heavy periods (menorrhagia), irregular cycles and extended periods, and painful periods (dysmenorrhoea), benefited from thyroid therapy. He confirmed the value of thyroid support by noting that the women who obtained symptom relief and subsequently discontinued their thyroid treatment, often suffered a reoccurrence of their menstrual symptoms. A return to thyroid medication, once more cleared the symptoms[4].

In 1964 a study by Scott and Mussey discussed 50 women with hypothyroidism. More than 50 per cent suffered menstrual symptoms and symptom relief was obtained following thyroid treatment[5]. A deficiency of thyroid hormones can cause heavy prolonged periods. Similar symptoms can develop following thyroid surgery for hyperthyroidism. The exact links between thyroid underactivity and menstrual symptoms have yet to be proven, however possible changes to blood viscosity and flow, and the thyroid's influence on the metabolism of the sex hormones are both implicated. The beneficial effects of thyroid therapy on women with menstrual irregularities have been demonstrated by trials and treatment over many years.

ANGELA'S STORY

At her consultation Angela described her condition as pre-menstrual tension, because she claimed to know what 'tension' was but did not know what a 'syndrome' felt like. She was 33 years old, with a good health record, married but without children. The only thing that marred her well-being was the four or five days of depression and moodiness that preceded every period. She claimed to have suffered PMS 'forever', but questioning revealed that the symptoms had commenced when she was a student around the age of 18 or 19.

She admitted that over recent years her pre-menstrual symptoms had been more varied and more severe, including an acute sugar craving, fatigue, a weight gain of 6–8lb, and a pounding headache. She had sought the advice of various therapists and with the help of a hypoglycaemic diet, specific vitamin and mineral supplements, plus capsules of blackcurrant seed oil (a good source of the omega-6 fatty acids) she was now left with only two symptoms that really concerned her. These symptoms were a black depression and irritability or general moodiness. Angela hastened to tell me that she was normally quite happy and non-moody, which contrasted with her pre-menstrual symptoms. Both she and her partner had learned to dread her monthly personality changes.

As the physical symptoms of fluid retention, headache and fatigue had cleared, Angela's GP had diagnosed clinical depression and prescribed an antidepressant drug.

Angela was not happy with this situation and consulted me to find out what a naturopath would diagnose, and if anything else could be done.

DIAGNOSIS

When questioning a patient at a consultation it is not always sufficient to ask them 'What is your problem?' or 'What are your symptoms?'. Rather it sometimes becomes necessary to ask leading questions. This is required because many patients do not regard certain symptoms as being significant, nor do they see them as being a health problem.

With mild hypothyroidism, symptoms are never confined to a four to five day time slot just before periods. Although as discussed earlier the thyroid is often implicated as one of the causes of PMS, any other symptoms would persist throughout the month.

With this in mind I asked Angela a standard series of questions that I ask with suspected mild hypothyroidism.

These being:

1   Is your energy at the same level of five years earlier?
2   Is your concentration as it was five years earlier?
3   Is your short-term memory as sharp as your long-term memory?
4   Do you experience any aches and pains or stiffness in muscles and joints?
5   When do you feel at your worst, on rising, after lunch or upon retiring?
6   Do you consider that you are a warm or cold person?
7   Do you suffer any digestive problems or constipation?
8   Have you had any recent blood tests for the blood fats in particular cholesterol?
9   How is your sex drive?
10   Are you a stressful person?

Angela's answers provided some very useful data. She was not so vital as she was five years earlier and her short-term memory was 'terrible'. She felt stiff and tired on waking and improved throughout the day. Her hands were always cold and she disliked the winter weather. She had suffered from constipation most of her life, but her sex drive was satisfactory.

Angela stated that she was only stressed for four or five days each month, and she had not had a blood test for many years.

Following this information gathering I requested a full thyroid screen and a morning temperature check.

The free T$_4$ was towards the bottom of the reference range and Angela's morning temperatures showed an average of 96.8°F (36°C).

TREATMENT

I prescribed thyroid glandular supplements and a general vitamin, mineral, and amino acid thyroid supplement.

At the three month review, Angela was feeling noticeably more vital and her moods and depression were beginning to lift. After six months her blood T₄ was increased by 20 per cent and she was almost free from symptoms. Although she still experienced a residual 'gloom' before periods, her overall energy and mood were much improved.

SUMMARY

In common with many other patients who suffer the symptoms of mild hypothyroidism, Angela commented that only after she had felt so much better, did she appreciate that she had been tired for several years. Many such symptoms are so deceptively slow in onset that patients assume they are caused by their age or 'modern stress', and tend for these reasons not to seek help.

If you suffer from PMS, as well as some of the other symptoms of hypothyroidism, it is well worth drawing together a symptom picture (see Part Two) and approaching your doctor or complementary practitioner.

CHAPTER SIX

'Why do I Ache?'

The Thyroid and Your Joints and Muscles

Having practised as an osteopath and naturopath for 36 years and treated chronic fatigue for more than 20 years, I have frequently seen hypothyroid patients experiencing symptoms of muscle and joint pain and stiffness. The links between an underactive thyroid and muscle–joint health are complex and controversial, yet the evidence that thyroid function influences muscles and joints has been well proven.

There has been a great deal of research over the last century which has attempted to establish a link between underactive thyroid and muscle-joint symptoms. I have summarized some of this research on pages 86–88. In this chapter I am going to address some of the common muscle–joint illnesses which have been successfully treated through hypothyroid medication. If you suffer from rheumatism, joint swelling, arthritis or any related problems use the information below – as well as the case histories – to build up an idea of whether you may have undiagnosed mild hypothyroidism.

Common Muscular–Joint Conditions

Carpal Tunnel Syndrome

This surprisingly common syndrome includes pins and needles (paraesthesia) in the hand or hands with numbness and occasional pain passing up the arm. The carpal tunnel is in the wrist and the symptoms can be caused by the pressure of the tissue congestion and fluid retention on the median nerve which passes through the tunnel. The thyroid is often a cause of these symptoms when it becomes underactive. Employment involving repeated specific hand movements or repetitive strain injury (RSI) can trigger or worsen the carpal tunnel symptoms.

Repetitive strain injury (RSI) cases are increasingly featured in the media. Particularly in the context of employee injury claims with large compensation payouts.

Work related injuries and symptoms are not new. Most manual employment whether brick-laying, gardening or cleaning, has been known to carry a risk of joint strain or more serious injuries.

The RSI concept however, defines symptoms in joints and muscles that have developed as a result of repetitive small scale – even light – use of a muscle group or limb.

Other names for RSI include work related upper limb disorder (WRULD), occupational overuse syndrome and cumulative trauma disorder.

The main group of workers who seem to suffer from RSI are keyboard operators. When I am consulted by patients suffering from RSI type symptoms, I always find that it is worthwhile doing a general health check, and thyroid function tests are usually included in such a review. With many cases of RSI it is quite possible that underlying ill health predisposes to the symptoms. Perhaps explaining why some people suffer RSI and others doing the same work are symptom-free.

Dupuytren's Contracture

This condition describes a painless progressive thickening and tightening of the tissues in the palm, or palms. This can cause the ring and little fingers to flex into the palm of the hand. This condition was seen as evidence of hypothyroidism as early as 1917 being described by McCarrison[3] (see page 86).

Muscular Rheumatism

The adverse influence of hypothyroidism on muscle strength and flexibility has been known for many years. The chief areas affected being the neck and shoulders, the lower back and lower legs. In severe hypothyroidism the loss of strength in the muscles of the neck and upper back can cause a forward slump of the posture (kyphosis) and a clumsy slow gait. General neck and back stiffness are typical symptoms of thyroid deficit. These symptoms being particularly pronounced upon waking. Cold, damp weather can worsen muscle conditions that are caused by hypothyroidism, and ease of bruising and muscle cramping are also common.

Although the symptoms may be similar to rheumatoid arthritis there is an absence of joint tenderness and swelling and the specific blood tests for arthritis are usually normal.

> Some confusion exists over the terms rheumatism and arthritis.
>
> Rheumatism describes a syndrome consisting of pain, inflammation and stiffness of any type of tissue but chiefly muscles, ligaments and joints.
>
> Arthritis more specifically defines inflammation of a joint or joints.
>
> When rheumatism is confined to the joints it is usually classified as arthritis.

The severity of muscular symptoms in hypothyroidism on waking has been likened to polymyalgia rheumatica, but without the characteristic blood picture of this complaint. Chronic shoulder stiffness is also a common feature of hypothyroidism.

All the above symptoms are exacerbated by the muscle fatigue, poor circulation and excess weight. Symptoms that are so typical in hypothyroidism.

Bursitis and Joint Swelling

The tissue congestion and fluid retention of hypothyroidism can cause synovial swellings, particularly in the knee joints.

> The synovial membrane refers to the joint lining that secretes the synovial fluid which serves to lubricate the joint. The fluid may accumulate in excessively painful amounts when a joint is injured e.g. bursitis of the knee.

This inflammation of the muscles can make people stiff and clumsy. These symptoms are worsened with rest, damp and cold. The blood test that indicates the presence of inflammation (erythrocyte sedimentation rate – or ESR) is frequently raised with hypothyroidism.

Fibromyalgia (Fibrositis)

Many patients suffering the symptoms of fibromyalgia have also been diagnosed as suffering from hypothyroidism. This thyroid link, however, is not always confirmed in laboratory tests for thyroid hormones, suggesting that either the normal range is being interpreted too rigidly, or the patient's conversion of T_4 to T_3 is not efficient (see page 181).

JOHN'S STORY

John's symptoms had baffled his doctor for two years. He was a retired engineer aged 66, who for many years had enjoyed good health, except for a chronic low back problem resulting from a road traffic accident 40 years ago.

THE CONSULTATION

When John consulted me, he complained of a worsening back problem in addition to the following symptoms:

*   Pain and weakness in the leg muscles
*   Leg cramp with walking (intermittent claudication)
*   Constipation
*   Poor wound healing with a tendency to easily bruise
*   Fibromyalgia type muscle pain across the neck and shoulders
*   General loss of energy
*   Very cold feet

After blood tests, scans and X-rays his doctor concluded that John suffered from fibromyalgia (fibrositis), caused by a lifelong tendency to spend too much time and effort looking after a very large garden.

John's weight, blood pressure, diet and sleeping habits were all quite normal and satisfactory. However, his average morning temperature was 97.6°F and his thyroid hormone levels were borderline, being towards the lower end of the normal range.

> John's symptoms did not fit exactly into a diagnosis of mild hypothyroidism. His temperature was only marginally low and he seemed quite alert, without anxiety or depression. This highlights the need to exercise clinical judgement with hypothyroidism and not to strictly rely on test results. It would have been an easy solution to diagnose John as a retired man who had worked too hard and played too hard.

THE TREATMENT

In spite of these doubts, I decided to treat him as a case of mild hypothyroidism. A programme of nutritional support including multi-minerals, proteins and vitamins was recommended. Also a course of thyroid glandular supplements. John was also encouraged to take up swimming and cycling and reduce his heavy gardening activities.

THE PROGRESS

Within six months his temperature had normalized and the blood thyroid hormones had increased. His spinal pain and claudication had noticeably improved.

Hypothyroidism does not always present a characteristic symptom-picture. Many factors can influence the variability of symptoms. These include:

* Family history
* Previous health history
* Past treatment and past surgery
* Duration of the symptoms
* Patient's age
* Patient's weight
* Occupation
* Stress factors
* Immune efficiency
* General human individuality

For this reason I believe that a diagnosis needs to be based on the clinical assessment of symptoms, the morning temperatures and the levels of the hormones that influence thyroid activity.

One of the main advantages of Naturopathic treatment, is the safety factor. A three to four month trial on glandular and/or supplements can be prescribed with the reassurance that side effects will not develop. Any past uncertainty over the accuracy of diagnosis can be set aside when the symptoms improve and the temperatures and blood readings slowly normalize.

John's case demonstrates once again the great variety in the symptom picture presented in mild hypothyroidism.

RESEARCH PAPERS

Dr W. M. Ord, who first defined myxoedema (severe hypothyroidism), described the rheumatic symptoms of his hypothyroid patients, these included swollen fingers and generalized thickening and stiffness of the joints[1]. Shortly after Ord's work in 1877, Sir Victor Horsley observed that removal of the thyroid glands of sheep lead to tissue thickening and fluid retention in the animals. This being reversed with thyroid treatment[2].

Robert McCarrison wrote a classic textbook in 1917, entitled *The Thyroid Gland in Health and Disease*. He observed that patients with underactive thyroids suffered from muscle and ligament contractions with subsequent stiffness and weakness. The areas mainly affected being the neck and shoulders, the abdominal muscles, the lower back and the calves and feet, pain, cramp and stiffness being typical symptoms, many of which were reversed when the thyroid was successfully treated[3].

In 1929, the *American Medical Journal* carried an article by Dr Loring T. Swain of Boston describing the treatment of 67 arthritic patients using whole desiccated animal thyroid. He noted the tendency of all arthritic patients to have a low metabolic rate. With treatment, his test patients all showed an increase in general vitality and circulation, with a subsequent reduction in the arthritic stiffness and pain[4].

During the programme he made a very interesting observation that 'clinical observance of thyroid symptoms is the best guide as a patient's metabolic rate is not a good indication'.

He concluded by stating that 'a low metabolic rate may be a pre-arthritic sign or that patients in the low metabolic group are those in whom arthritis develops'.

Significantly it has been known for many years that arthritic patients are prone to infections and fatigue. Chronic stress usually features in their health history.

In a paper by D. N. Golding published in 1970, a group of patients with a variety of muscle-joint symptoms were tested for rheumatoid arthritis, gout and osteoarthritis. The testing included blood tests and X-rays, the results all showed normal readings. However, hypothyroidism was suspected when the patients also presented symptoms of fatigue, body coldness, overweight and a slow pulse. Specific thyroid blood tests plus total cholesterol measurements were used to confirm hypothyroidism in many of the patients in the group. The patients' symptoms also included one or more of the following:

* muscle weakness
* pain and stiffness
* carpal tunnel syndrome
* muscle cramps.

The paper's summary stated that: 'In all cases the symptoms were alleviated by the administration of thyroid hormone' and concluded that 'hypothyroidism should be considered in the differential diagnosis of patients' presenting with rheumatism'[5].

Another worthwhile paper entitled 'Musculoskeletal Symptoms as a Presenting Sign of Long-standing Hypothyroidism' served to show the influence of thyroid function on muscles and joints. It appeared in the *Israeli Journal of Medical Sciences* in 1987. Dr Krupsky and his co-authors stated that 'the cases presented illustrate that hypothyroidism can lead to the development of a variety of muscular rheumatic and dermatologic syndromes'[6].

Dermatology refers to the study of the skin and the diagnosis and treatment of skin conditions or pathologies.

This reference presented two worthwhile pieces of evidence.

1   The blood of the hypothyroid test patients showed excessively high levels of muscle enzymes as a result of the enzymes being released from damaged muscles. These enzyme levels normalized following thyroid hormone therapy.

2   No evidence was found of a systemic auto-immune process, indicating that any changes to muscle tissue were entirely the result of the thyroid deficiency. There was also a full recovery of all the musculo-skeletal symptoms when the patients' thyroids were treated.

The paper concluded that 'hypothyroidism should be seriously considered in the differential diagnosis of patients presenting with connective tissue symptoms'.

The dictionary defines differential diagnosis as 'the distinguishing between two or more diseases with similar symptoms by systematically comparing their signs and symptoms'.

Connective tissue supports and binds other body tissue and organs together. Diseases of the connective tissue include lupus (SLE), rheumatoid arthritis, rheumatic fever and certain skin and blood circulation disorders.

Muscle–Joint Pain and the Adrenal Glands

In the 1940s doctors discovered a hormone produced from the adrenal glands called cortisone. Many doctors were convinced this could lead to a cure for arthritis. Unfortunately it was later shown that the side effects from corticosteroids (cortisone and related hormones) were worse than the symptoms being treated. Moreover, patients showed similar side effects from the corticosteroid treatment as those who suffer from hypothyroidism. These symptoms included the familiar picture of weight increase, depression, skin conditions and bruising. Corticosteroids can clearly be shown to have a depressing effect on the thyroid.

> Pregnenolone is a steroid hormone which does not cause any side effects. It is not, however, as potent as cortisone. Pregnenolone has a proven value in treating joint pain and inflammation.

Studies have shown that arthritic patients with hypothyroidism do not respond well to steroid therapy, this being reversed however when their thyroids are balanced with treatment this and other research lead Broda Barnes in 1970 to combine thyroid and corticosteroid treatment with selected patients suffering from arthritis and rheumatism.[7]

The prescription included low dosage prednisone (cortisone) coupled with thyroid medication. Over a four year period, Barnes treated in excess of 200 patients with this combination therapy, all of whom obtained symptom relief. Barnes believed that the key to his successful, side effect free combination schedule was to determine the optimum dosage of thyroid medication (based on the patient's morning temperatures) and then prescribe the low dosage prednisone. The thyroid depressing side effects of the prednisone are then minimized.

I do not prescribe adrenal or thyroid hormones, however, I do prescribe combination adrenal and thyroid glandular supplements for arthritis and similar illnesses. I also recommend DHEA and pregnenolone for a range of muscle–joint conditions. (More information on this system of treatment can be found in chapter ten.)

Summary

All the evidence and the clinical research and experience of many doctors and other practitioners points to the thyroid as being a major component in causing joint–muscle pain and stiffness. Underactivity of this vital gland can cause a host of symptoms and also influence other endocrine glands and body systems.

Unlike many illnesses the signs and symptoms of arthritis and rheumatism can be quite accurately diagnosed and monitored. Joint pain reduction and improved muscle–joint flexibility can result from a combined adrenal–thyroid treatment approach. Other elements in a treatment strategy should include the immune system, protein, vitamin and mineral status, body weight, the stress-effects and parallel illnesses and treating the many different joint disorders that affect our mobility and health.

SIMON'S STORY

Simon could only sleep on his back. For six months prior to consulting me his painful shoulders had prevented comfortable side-lying. The shoulder stiffness and pain was accompanied by stiffness in both wrists and in particular pain and stiffness in the thumb joints. All these symptoms were much worse on waking, or with prolonged sitting or driving.

Simon's wife now routinely helped him to dress, for his shoulder pain and stiffness prevented him raising his arms and putting a coat on without pain. As a full time writer he was finding that working on his word processor was becoming increasingly painful, and he could only write comfortably with a pen for five to 10 minutes.

Simon had undergone major surgery for a benign stomach tumour two years earlier. The removal of half of his stomach had caused him to lose weight and he subsequently developed iron deficient anaemia. Over the following 18 months his anaemia cleared and his weight normalized, however, he remained fatigued and depressed and his motivation to write was seriously reduced. Other symptoms included poor concentration and poor short-term memory and a total loss of sex drive. However, his main concern was the increasing pain and stiffness in his shoulders and hands.

EXAMINATION

Th examination revealed chronic muscle tension and tenderness in the neck and upper spine with shoulder movement reduced by at least 50 per cent. Simon's hand grip strength was poor and although no swelling was evident, his hands and wrists were sensitive to pressure and movement. Simon's lifestyle was excellent, he enjoyed a good balanced diet and avoided smoking. He only drank 10 to 15 units of wine each week. The only medication or supplements he took was a low dose multi-mineral. Prior to the stomach operation he had enjoyed very good health. The pressures of his frequent editorial deadlines, coupled with the recent fatigue and joint pain were now causing him considerable stress and anxiety. Simon's only income came from his writing and he had lost or cancelled several projects while he was convalescing.

DIAGNOSIS

As Simon was 55 years old I felt it wise to request X-rays of his hands and shoulders to check for osteoarthritis. A full blood screen was also requested and I asked Simon to measure his morning temperatures for three days.

The X-rays were clear with no sign of excessive joint wear or arthritis and nothing significant showed with the blood test results. I concluded that Simon was probably suffering from non-specific fibromyalgia with muscular rheumatism. However, his morning temperature averaged 97.2°F (36.2°C) and I requested a full thyroid profile. His thyroid hormones showed a low grade hypothyroidism.

TREATMENT

In addition to osteopathic treatment and local acupuncture, I pre-scribed thyroid and adrenal glandular support and increased Simon's mineral supplements. I also advised him to take omega 3 fish oil cap-sules to treat any joint inflammation. Although progress was slow, within six months Simon was almost symptom-free. His joints being more mobile and with a general increase in energy and optimism. A second thyroid test six months after the consultation showed a 30 per cent increase in his free T₄ (thyroxine) level and his morning tempera-tures were averaging 97.6°F.

Sometime after discussing progress with Simon he mentioned that he was convinced before his surgery that he had stomach cancer. We cannot measure the effects of this type of stress, but adrenal exhaus-tion with hypofunction of the whole endocrine axis, including the thy-roid, can result from chronic stress. Major surgery, with the subsequent weight loss and anaemia all served to reduce Simon's muscle health and adrenal efficiency. This produced a glandular chain-reaction effect that can so often lead to mild hypothyroidism. Once the vicious circle of fatigue, joint pain, anxiety and more fatigue is established, only accu-rate diagnosis and appropriate treatment can prevent the problem becoming irreversible. When this stage is reached the X-rays and blood tests are rarely 'clear'.

When questioning arthritic patients on their past health, I often hear a familiar history of overweight, fatigue and stress that points to a missed hypothyroid condition.

CHAPTER SEVEN

'Can my Fatigue Affect my Heart?'

The Thyroid Gland and Your Heart

Although this chapter will mainly concern you if you are over 50 years of age, it is also worth reading this chapter if you are younger; some young patients have been known to develop circulation problems caused as a result of hypothyroidism.

The heart and circulation are adversely affected by a low grade hypothyroidism in various ways.

The Thyroid and Your Heart Rate

When the metabolic rate is slowed down, the heart rate will also slow down. Consequently, when the heart rhythm is disturbed the heart becomes inefficient, and tissue congestion and fluid retention can occur. This can lead to swelling of the ankles (oedema), and shortage of breath (dyspnoea).

The Thyroid Connection

As early as the 1890s, researchers observed that removal of the thyroid in test animals caused the development of atherosclerosis and tissue fluid congestion. Up until the 1950s it was standard surgical practice to remove the whole thyroid gland when they treated patients with very large goitres. This was in spite of the evidence that the operation invariably caused myxoedema and degeneration of the blood vessels throughout the body. The coronary arteries that supplied the heart did not escape this destructive outcome.

> Dr Stephen Langer in his book *Solved the Riddle of Illness*, makes an interesting observation. 'A low voltage reading on the electrocardiogram reveals the status of the thyroid gland more accurately than many common blood tests for thyroid function, as many doctors have discovered'.[1]

Circulation Changes

Other complications of a deficient thyroid's effect on the heart include a general weakening of the heart muscle, and more specifically a condition known as coronary atherosclerosis. This defines a narrowing or a 'furring-up' of the blood vessels that supply fuel and oxygen to the heart. Cramping of the heart muscle following effort (angina) can result from this condition. When the fluid retention includes the fibrous sac that surrounds the heart (the pericardium), there occurs a rapid increase of pressure around the heart. This is known as pericardial effusion, which is seen as an early sign of congenital heart failure.

Other circulation symptoms made worse by thyroid disease can include Raynaud's phenomenon, cramping of the leg muscles when walking (intermittent claudication), body coldness, restless leg syndrome (involuntary leg movements when lying down, especially at night), bruising, chilblains, poor wound healing, reduced perspiration, slow pulse and raised blood pressure. Iron deficient anaemia can also result from hypothyroidism. The red cell production in the bone marrow is reduced as a result of the abnormally low body temperature that occurs with a depressed thyroid. This can also cause a reduction of tissue oxygen. Anaemia can further diminish the metabolic rate and the body temperature, establishing a vicious circle of fatigue and body coldness.

> The Swiss physicians Lidsky and Kottman demonstrated that blood clotting is accelerated in hypothyroidism. The blood viscosity increases as the metabolism slows. The combination of narrow, hardened arteries and the existence of blood clots can be fatal. They were also able to show that the clotting function normalized with successful thyroid treatment.[2]

The Cholesterol Controversy

Many physicians consider that a diet high in cholesterol-rich foods and animal fat can cause a heart attack.

This view is difficult to substantiate when presented with historical evidence, and the evidence obtained from current comparative studies of different national diets.

In eighteenth century Europe over 90 per cent of the population were agricultural workers. Their diet consisted of dairy products, meat, cured meats, lard and milk. The farmers in particular were well fed on high cholesterol foods, yet heart disease was a great rarity. In the medical textbooks of the time, heart disease was described as a cause of death for the very elderly, not as a disease.

African herdsmen (Somali and Masai tribesmen) often live on a high meat, high animal fat diet, yet heart disease in these groups is almost unknown.

Man has eaten animal fats for thousands of years. It does seem unlikely that these fats now constitute a major cause of twentieth century coronary heart disease.

Significantly, the total fat consumption in the USA has only increased by 12 per cent in 70 years. This increase consists chiefly of fish and vegetable oils.

Around 50 per cent of those who die as a result of heart disease have a normal blood cholesterol.

Heart Attacks – A Historical View

Heart attacks in Western nations have increased tenfold over the last 60 years.

The main cause of death before the Second World War was infectious diseases, which accounted for approximately 50 per cent of all deaths, with tuberculosis being the number one killer. However by the 1970s deaths by infections had fallen by 60 per cent. Autopsy evidence confirmed that in the 1930s death from infections accounted for 426 deaths per 1,000 autopsies, whilst deaths from heart attacks only accounted for six to eight deaths per 1,000 autopsies. Heart attacks were rare, but with the introduction of antibiotics in the 1940s fewer people died young of infections and the average age of death over the age of 50 years increased by 20 per cent in 40 years.

> Percentage of total population dying over the age of 50
> years in 1930 – 47%
> Percentage of total population dying over the age of 50
> years in 1970 – 67%

WHY THE INCREASE IN HEART DISEASE?

So people were living longer but dying from different causes. The question that needed to be answered was, 'Why did the patients surviving the infections as a result of the invention of antibiotics, become prone to heart disease in later life?' Was it simply that they were living longer and developing coronary heart disease as part of the ageing process?

Other factors have been blamed, including sugar intake, smoking, modern stress, lack of exercise and obesity. However, the significant statistic is that in one generation the title of the chief killer had switched from tuberculosis to heart disease.

It has been argued since the 1930s that hypothyroidism raises the blood cholesterol and hyperthyroidism lowers the cholesterol. Some researchers were so convinced of the predictability of the thyroid–cholesterol see-saw that they regarded the blood cholesterol level as a diagnostic tool to identify a depressed thyroid. Furthermore, they considered that the value of any treatment on the thyroid could be assessed by the corresponding decrease in a patient's cholesterol level. Experiments have conclusively shown that eating cholesterol rich foods (e.g. eggs) does not necessarily increase the blood cholesterol. The liver is designed to reduce production of cholesterol when we eat sufficient, and when our intake of cholesterol is low, the liver cells increase production. The cholesterol level of our blood does not therefore accurately reflect the amount of cholesterol we consume.

Apart from an underactive thyroid, what else can raise our blood cholesterol? Heredity plays a major role, stress, obesity, high blood pressure, smoking, high sugar intake, insufficient exercise and a raised blood uric acid (as in gout), are all contributive factors. As the liver produces up to 60 per cent of the blood cholesterol, a toxic liver can also raise the blood level.

What is Cholesterol?

Total cholesterol is split into HDL and LDL. HDL or high density lipoprotein is the good or beneficial fraction, LDL or low density lipoprotein can be seen as the bad or harmful fraction. This means that a raised HDL and a lowered LDL can reduce the risk of heart disease. Cholesterol does not mix with water, and the transport of cholesterol is achieved by linking it with the lipoproteins. These consist of a combination of fats and proteins. The functions of HDL and LDL serve to demonstrate their effects on human health. HDL assists in removal of excess cholesterol for processing and elimination by the liver, whilst LDL transports cholesterol and fat directly to the body cells, leading to a possible excess. The key to heart protection by increasing the HDL to LDL ratio lies in the correct combination of diet and exercise. Tobacco should be avoided in addition to the following changes:

1   Reduce animal fats (saturated fats) and eat fish two to three times weekly. These should be cold water fish (see section on EFA's in Appendix A).
2   Reduce weight.
3   Identify and treat any thyroid imbalance.
4   Exercise regularly (first discuss this with your physician).
5   Specific nutritional supplements are also of value – see pages 148-149.

What Use is Cholesterol?

For many years cholesterol has received a quite unnecessary bad press. It has been unfairly blamed for a host of cardiovascular symptoms including the dramatic increase in coronary heart disease that has occurred over the last 30 years.

Perhaps it would be worthwhile to remind readers of the value of cholesterol. It is a fat-soluble, steroid alcohol found in animal fats, oils and egg yolk. Cholesterol is widely distributed in the body, being found chiefly in the bile, blood, brain tissue, the liver, the kidneys, the adrenal glands and the fatty casing of nerves.

> Eggs are now available (in America) that are from hens whose feed is enriched with omega-3 oils. Studies have shown that eating two of these eggs each day can lower triglycerides and increase the HDL cholesterol.

Its functions include fatty acid transport and absorption, and the synthesis of vitamin D on the skin's surface. It also acts as a precursor for the adrenal hormones (e.g. cortisone, DHEA and aldosterone) and the sex hormones (progesterone, oestrogen and testosterone). It is also the main constituent of bile salts.

It is found almost exclusively in foods of animal origin but it is worth noting that around 60 per cent of the cholesterol in our blood is synthesized directly by the liver.

> It has been demonstrated that when cholesterol free diets have been followed for several weeks the blood cholesterol has actually risen as a result of its increased production by the liver.

TRIGLYCERIDES

These substances, which have caused a great deal of public confusion constitute the main fat found in our blood, and not cholesterol. Triglycerides are produced by the liver from carbohydrates. Most animal and vegetable fats consist of triglycerides. Increased amounts found in the blood are significant in many diseases including diabetes, high blood pressure and heart disease. The modern high sugar diet is implicated in high levels, which can lead to thickening of the blood. With this in mind, I usually check the triglycerides level of patients who show mild hypothyroidism. The combination of a raised LDL, raised cholesterol, hypothyroidism and raised triglycerides calls for prompt and thorough treatment.

The Thyroid and High Blood Pressure

Many hypothyroid patients suffer with raised blood pressure, this can contribute to coronary heart disease and stroke. In spite of the increasing frequency of this problem the causes are still not fully understood, in fact up to 90 per cent of patients are diagnosed with essential or idiopathic hypertension. 'Essential' in this context means simply, 'for which no cause can be found'. Perhaps one of the unknown causes is hypothyroidism.

At first sight the notion of a raised blood pressure does not sit easily into the underactive thyroid symptom picture. We tend to associate underactivity with reduced function and low levels, circulation and immune deficiency, loss of muscle strength, poor concentration and memory, reduced sex drive and many other similar symptoms. The chronic fatigue that often accompanies a low thyroid function, would normally be thought to be caused by low blood pressure, as with anaemia and adrenal exhaustion. So why, you may ask, does the blood pressure tend so often to rise with a low thyroid?

What is Blood Pressure?

The two readings taken when measuring the blood pressure reflect the arterial pressure. When the heart beats the reading taken is called the systolic pressure or higher reading, and when the heart rests it is termed the diastolic pressure or the lower reading. The pressure will constantly change with rest, stress, activity and eating. The ideal resting blood pressure is a systolic pressure of 100–150 and a diastolic pressure of 60-90. A single reading well below or well above these figures is not considered significant. However, continuous readings over a period of time of a systolic below 100 suggests hypotension (low blood pressure), and over 150 suggests hypertension (high blood pressure).

As you may be aware the blood pressure can be checked in less than a minute. Unfortunately many patients become stressed and tense when they visit a physician, and an artificially high blood pressure can be the result. This 'white coat' hypertension can provide false information. For this reason 24 hour monitoring of the blood pressure, with automatic checks every 30 minutes, is being increasingly requested to obtain an accurate overview of a patient's blood pressure pattern. This type of assessment provides fascinating and valuable information, showing the effects of rest, stress, eating and work on a person's blood pressure over the 24 hour period. Unfortunately a person may not be aware that their blood pressure is too high. I have seen patients with figures in excess of 180 without any symptoms being present. Even when symptoms are experienced – and these can include headaches, fatigue and dizziness – they are so common to many other health problems that hypertension is not always suspected.

The Thyroid Effect

The influence of an underactive thyroid on the blood pressure can be seen in five ways:

1   A reduction in the blood supply to the kidneys can raise the blood pressure. This can occur in hypothyroidism as a result of atherosclerosis of the kidney blood vessels.

2   Surgery to treat thyroid enlargement (goitre) has shown that the blood pressure increases in proportion to the amount of thyroid gland removed.

3   Operations to remove the thyroid (thyroidectomy) can cause hypertension, or worsen an existing tendency.

4   There is evidence available to show that patients who are successfully treated for hypothyroidism do not have high blood pressure. Furthermore, if they have high blood pressure before treatment, the thyroid therapy reduces the pressure without the need for anti-hypertension drugs.

5   The increased body weight, fluid retention and raised blood cholesterol that occurs with hypothyroidism, can all contribute to high blood pressure.

Although many cases of hypertension are not related to thyroid underactivity, it is a link that should be investigated. Raised blood pressure has been likened to revving up a motor car engine. It wastes energy, stresses the system and may damage the walls of the blood vessels. Some researchers believe that high blood pressure can contribute to arterial narrowing by increasing the risk of blood clotting around the sites where the vessel lining has been weakened.

CHAPTER EIGHT

'Why Won't my Skin Clear Up?'

The Thyroid Gland and Your Skin

Mild hypothyroidism can have a harmful effect on your skin. A low thyroid function reduces circulation to your skin causing it to become cold and dry. In addition, when the circulation is impaired, the nutrition and elimination of your skin is affected and local bacterial infections causing inflammation and sepsis can develop. All this suggests that skin disorders are an underestimated symptom of hypothyroidism, and if you have problem skin it is well worth investigating the possiblity of a underactive thyroid.

Common Skin Conditions

Boils and Carbuncles

Infection around a hair follicle or sebaceous gland can lead to pustule development with swelling and pain. If multiple drainage points result, a very painful and large carbuncle can occur. Although boils can also be caused and aggravated by diabetes, stress, anaemia and general toxaemia, I consider that a blood thyroid test is always worth requesting with such conditions. Other causative factors include zinc, vitamin A, and essential fatty acids deficiency (particularly omega-6) and poor personal hygiene.

Impetigo, Cellulitis and Erysipelas

These are all linked to streptococcal infections. Although these skin conditions can all respond to thorough naturopathic treatment, there is often an underlying mild hypothyroidism, which can so easily be missed. Aside from the poor circulation to the skin often found in hypothyroidism, there is also an accumulation under the skin of a substance known as mucin. When Ord first defined under-activity of the thyroid as myxoedema in 1877, he made use of the Greek work for mucin which is myx. Mucin consists of compounds known as mucopolysaccharides. These compounds accumulate in body tissue, particularly the skin, when the thyroid function is depressed. Significantly, an excess of mucopolysaccharides can be reduced following successful thyroid treatment.

> Mucin is the chief constituent of mucus. This excess of mucin accounts for the general sluggishness of muscles that accompanies low thyroid function. The mucous membranes are also affected by the mucin increase, leading to conjunctivitis, rhinitis, bronchitis and cystitis. All these conditions have been known to accompany hypothyroidism.

Acne

This common skin problem is typically attributed to an excess of testosterone. The surge of the male hormone at puberty is said to explain the incidence of acne in teenage boys. However, I find that many acne sufferers (particularly the older patients) have a low thyroid function and benefit from thyroid treatment. I also look closely at the patient's omega-3 status and the need for vitamin A, the B complex vitamins and zinc. A Mediterranean diet is appropriate for acne, with the total avoidance of sugar and all forms of cows' milk in favour of fruit, salads and vegetables, garlic, olive oil and seafood.

The widespread influence and the powerful role of the thyroid gland in skin health has been demonstrated clearly and conclusively in various ways. Laboratory animals show rapid deterioration in their health following removal of their thyroids. They shiver with cold and move as if exhausted or aged. The quality of their fur deteriorates and they become prone to chest infections and heart weakness.

TESSA'S STORY

Tessa had been prescribed amitriptyline by her doctor. He considered that she suffered from clinical depression. I considered that she suffered from profound unhappiness and a total loss of self-esteem. The cause was acne. Tessa was aged 35, and she had suffered from severe acne since her puberty at 12 years of age.

When she consulted me, I saw a slim, elegant young woman, whose face was covered with suppurating spots and blemishes. Her other symptoms included muscle stiffness on waking, cold hands and feet, and chronic candidiasis and cystitis. The latter being caused by frequent courses of antibiotics prescribed unsuccessfully for her acne. Tessa also lacked energy and found it hard to concentrate. Her past treatments, in addition to antibiotics, included many different diets, various creams, multi-vitamins and minerals, progesterone therapy, acupuncture, herbalism and homoeopathy. Although she had experienced temporary remissions, no lasting cure had been achieved and her skin had never completely cleared in 23 years. Tessa also suffered repeated winter colds and a very distressing allergic rhinitis triggered by house dust, cigarette smoke, animal fur, and seasonal pollen count surges. Blood tests had revealed 'nothing unusual'.

Although her diet seemed adequate I asked Tessa to list her complete intake of food and drink for seven days. I also requested a detailed list of her food supplements and any current medication.

> When I first began to practise I habitually asked patients to outline for me a typical day's diet. However, after some years it became obvious to me that many patients were describing a stereotype 'ideal diet', that did not accurately reflect their true pattern of eating.
>
> I now ask for full details of the food and drink consumed over a five or seven day period. Including times of eating, amounts, snacks etc. – in fact everything that passes their lips. This gastronomic diary can be quite revealing and certainly a lot more reliable than a 'typical day's menu'.

I also requested various blood tests including a thyroid profile, a mineral profile, and a test for essential fatty acids. Tessa was asked to check her morning temperatures.

The results showed a borderline hypothyroidism, a raised total cholesterol and LDL cholesterol, and an omega-3 fatty acid deficiency. Her mineral tests showed low levels of zinc, magnesium and iron. Although it was tempting to test for candidiasis, I considered that the condition could be assumed as a result of Tessa's history of antibiotics. I placed any further tests on hold, including a leaky gut test (PEG 400) and a food intolerance ELISA test, and awaited results with the thyroid, mineral and essential fatty acid (EFA) treatment.

I recommended that Tessa should follow a Mediterranean diet and advised her to totally avoid cows' milk foods and drinks, sugar and alcohol. She was prescribed raw glandular thyroid, a multi-mineral, a vitamin B complex, and a high dosage omega-3 EFAs; beta carotene and other antioxidants were also included.

The local or topical treatment of the acne spots can be disappointing. However, I have found that the use of Tea Tree oil may sometimes be very rewarding.

Tea Tree describes a family of Australian plants numbering over 300 varieties. The only plant with any medicinal properties is called Melaleuca alternifolia. The method of use is to wash the face well using Tea Tree oil soap and then to apply the oil with a finger or cotton bud directly to the acne spots twice daily. Another method is to add six drops of the pure oil to a little warm water and rinse the face two or three times daily.

Calendular cream and soap is also worth trying, and evening primrose oil, aloe vera gel and slippery elm ointment are all recommended.

A recent blood test has shown an improvement in Tessa's mineral status, the omega-3, EFAs and the thyroid function. After four months of treatment, her skin showed an approximate 50 per cent improvement. At the time of writing she is still under treatment, and although further treatment is required and her candidiasis will need to be treated, I feel sure that her acne and other symptoms will eventually be resolved. Tessa's case highlights just how severely an underfunctioning thyroid can affect skin health. Her case also shows the multi-causative pattern of many diseases and the value of treating the whole person, and not simply the symptoms.

Eczema

This condition is linked to food intolerances, and stress, yet many sufferers also show symptoms of a poorly functioning thyroid. The characteristic itching (pruritis) and scaling with dryness is typical of hypothyroidism. The combination of food sensitivities, and the tendency to poor infection control and inflammation that occurs in hypothyroidism, clearly demonstrates the role that the thyroid plays in causing eczema.

Psoriasis

Psoriasis is a skin condition characterized by the formation of reddish spots and patches covered with silvery scales. Psoriasis is a stubborn and complex skin condition. There are many types and no two patients are alike. The dry, scaly skin symptoms that occur are typical of the hypothyroid effect. I find it worthwhile checking the thyroid with psoriasis, however, I must admit that thyroid treatment is not a cure-all. Food intolerances, alcohol, the blood fats and adrenal exhaustion can all play a part in causing psoriasis. There is rarely one cause for this problem, but thyroid deficiency can play a major role.

Although psoriasis usually gives a dry, flaky appearance to the skin, localized pustular psoriasis looks very different. This particularly distressing form of psoriasis can usually be seen on the palms of the hands and the soles of the feet. It causes swelling, blisters, pustules and great discomfort.

MIKE'S STORY

Mike had suffered with psoriasis for 40 years. The characteristic crusty, scaly lesions being chiefly on the knees, elbows and back. His skin flexibility was so poor that flexion of the joints caused the skin to crack and bleed.

Mike also complained of a number of other symptoms. These included chronic fatigue, tinnitus, poor hearing, vertigo, migraines and a poor sense of smell and taste. Also neck and back pain, stiffness and raised blood pressure. In his own words he 'felt like death in the mornings' – and never really felt warm.

As a child he had suffered from chronic recurring tonsilitis and middle ear infections up to the age of 25, when his tonsils were finally removed. His hair had begun to turn grey at the age of 12.

He had experienced bouts of depression for many years, which fuelled his lack of self-confidence, and contributed to his short-term attention span and poor memory.

PAST TREATMENT

Mike had tried very hard to solve his health problems. An ear–nose–throat consultant had prescribed a hearing aid and numerous courses of antibiotics over several years. Mike had self-prescribed homoeopathic remedies and when he came to see me he admitted to taking a battery of vitamin and mineral supplements. The only skin relief obtained, however, was following the occasional use of steroid creams, unfortunately the skin rapidly worsened after their use was discontinued.

Mike's family history revealed that his father was a lifelong sufferer of psoriasis, and perceptive deafness featured in his mother's family. Upon examination it became evident that the psoriasis was not Mike's only skin problem. His whole skin surface was very dry and grey, with the characteristic loss of eyebrow hair and poor nail health that has been linked with thyroid dysfunction.

A full blood profile test showed nothing abnormal, but the thyroid function tests revealed a low level of thyroid hormone.

When a patient presents many symptoms and an underactive thyroid is diagnosed, it is tempting for a doctor to attribute 'all' the symptoms to the thyroid inefficiency. Occasionally this can be the case, but my own rule is to first treat and normalize the thyroid function and then carefully reassess any remaining symptoms.

Mild hypothyroidism can adversely influence nutrient absorption, cholesterol levels in the blood and anaemia. It cannot, however, be assumed that all thyroid-induced problems are curable with thyroid treatment. This particularly applies to long-term imbalances and deficiencies. The underactive thyroid may be a patient's central disorder, but secondary and associated health problems and symptoms may also require treatment. For example, a patient's vitamin B_{12} reserves may need to be replenished with the use of intramuscular vitamin B_{12} injections, or a high blood cholesterol may necessitate an anti-cholesterol diet and supplement programme.

To return to Mike, his basal temperature showed an average figure of 96°F (35.5°C). His blood pressure was raised and his weight was an acceptable 170lb. His age at consultation was 54.

TREATMENT

A full nutritional programme was designed for Mike – including thyroid glandular extract – with the aims of immune support, improved skin health and fatigue reduction. The latter was particularly helped by a course of vitamin B_{12} injections. The psoriasis improved about 75 per cent with the additional help of various herbal creams (I have found the Exorex range of banana based products of special value).

As we have seen in this chapter an underactive thyroid can have a damaging effect on your skin. Skin disorders are not only suffered by the young, but many people continue – or start – to suffer from acne, psoriasis or eczema throughout adulthood. If Mike's case sounds familiar, or if you suffer from a skin disorder which has persistently refused to respond to treatment, use Part Two to draw up a symptom picture and begin to assess whether you may suffer from undiagnosed hypothyroidism.

Diabetes and Hypothyroidism

In his book *Hypothyroidism* Broda Barnes reports several very useful statistics, including '...77 per cent of deaths in diabetes are due to blood vessel disease of one type or another'. He also states that 'many diabetics do, in fact, have low thyroid function'[1].

Dr Eaton noted in 1954 that 'hypothyroidism was frequent in diabetics, more so than the nondiabetic population'[2].

Significantly, all the complications that develop as a result of diabetes also occur in hypothyroidism without diabetes. These symptoms influence the nervous system, muscles, eyes, kidneys, joints and blood vessels.

Obesity is seen as one of the causes of diabetes and over 60 per cent of hypothyroid patients are overweight. The effect of hypothyroidism on the speed of digestion, the reduction in stomach acid and the pancreatic enzymes, plus the slow transit time and poor absorption rate that occurs with a depressed thyroid, can cause any blood sugar testing for diabetes to be unreliable.

A report in 1968 showed an apparent 50 per cent incidence of diabetes in 132 eskimos who were tested with glucose tolerance tests. As diabetes was at the time very rare amongst eskimos the test was repeated, but with the glucose being injected instead of taken by mouth. No diabetes showed in the second test. The slow glucose absorption in the first test that showed as false diabetes was considered to be caused by mild hypothyroidism.[3] To quote Broda Barnes 'Basal temperature testing in the Arctic Circle would be very interesting'.

I find that low thyroid function is more frequently found in diabetics than in non-diabetics. It is also worth remembering that although insulin may provide adequate control of the blood sugar levels, it does nothing to reduce the secondary symptoms of diabetes. A thyroid check, including basal temperatures measurements is therefore a wise step for diabetics.

Infections and Hypothyroidism

There is a strong connection between an underactive thyroid and susceptibility to infection. Laboratory tests have shown that when the thyroids of young rabbits are removed, the animals usually die of pneumonia. Before they die, however, they suffer repeated respiratory and other types of infections.

As we age our thyroid hormone levels reduce. It is no coincidence that many of the symptoms that are caused by an underactive thyroid are similar to the symptoms of ageing. These include reduced stamina, muscle and joint stiffness and pain, poor memory, reduced sex drive, hair loss, slow speech and poor hearing. With ageing and thyroid deficiency there is also a tendency to develop more infections.

To return to the rabbits; Dr Max Lurie wrote a paper dealing with the incidence of tuberculosis (TB) in two different types of rabbits[4]. The two breeds were infected with TB yet one breed developed TB while the other breed remained uninfected. It was then discovered that the non-TB breed were inherently hyperthyroid, whilst the breed that succumbed to TB were inherently hypothyroid. In other words the thyroid hormones exerted a powerful protective role against the TB bacteria. Thyroid hormones stimulate the production of lymphocytes. These white cells attack viruses, bacteria and other foreign substances. Our ability to successfully fight infections is therefore in part influenced by our thyroid health. Many physicians and research workers believe that chronic mild hypothyroidism explains why some people suffer only the occasional infection, yet others suffer repeated infections of every type. Significantly those who are prone to repeated infections are also prone to post-viral fatigue and a poor resistance to cold weather.

Although stress, insufficient sleep, poor nutrition and a poor family history can all lower our resistance to infections, depressed thyroid function can be a major influence.

PART TWO

Now you have read about some common symptoms of mild hypothyroidism which are frequently misdiagnosed or dismissed, it is time to look specifically at diagnosing your hypothyroidism and overcoming the condition through treatment.

Through using both home and medical diagnostic techniques you can begin to assess whether you may have an underactive thyroid. I will help you pull together a symptom picture which you should then present to a doctor or complementary practitioner experienced in thyroid disorders.

I will also show you how to diagnose fatigue and assess other illnesses which cause tiredness and lethargy.

Through diet, supplements and medical treatment you can recover your natural vitality, weight and well-being. Lifestyle changes, professional support, and simply understanding your condition, will return you to health.

CHAPTER NINE

Diagnosing Your Mild Hypothyroidism

There are three main strategies for assessing whether your fatigue is due to an underactive thyroid. These are:

A   Careful assessment of your signs and symptoms.
B   Taking your own body temperature after waking.
C   Asking your doctor or health practitioner to conduct laboratory tests.

In this chapter I will show you how to complete each of these three strategies.

Readers may be confused over the definitions of 'signs' and 'symptoms'. In medicine, symptoms are subjective sensations experienced by the patient, and include pain, sickness, coldness, stiffness etc. Signs are objective clues, or such evidence perceptible to the examining doctor. Examples are bruising, pallor, limping, skin lesions etc. So pain may be a symptom but a tendency to blush easily would be a sign. There may occasionally be a certain

> amount of overlapping of signs and symptoms, but the definitions generally hold true.

Strategy A: How Severe are Your Symptoms?

Although you may be diagnosed with mild hypothyroidism, the symptoms you may suffer can feel quite severe. I have seen many patients with all the evidence to suggest only a mild thyroid deficiency but who are suffering terribly from fatigue, depression or muscle pain.

Basic Questions to Ask Yourself

Before going further it is worth looking over the top 10 questions I ask my patients when I suspect mild hypothyroidism.

1   Is your energy at the same level as five years earlier?
2   Is your concentration as it was five years earlier?
3   Is your short-term memory as sharp as your long-term memory?
4   Do you experience any aches and pains or stiffness in muscles and joints?
5   When do you feel at your worst, on rising, after lunch or upon retiring?
6   Do you consider that you are a warm or cold person?
7   Do you suffer any digestive problems or constipation?
8   Have you had any recent blood tests for the blood fats, in particular cholesterol?
9   How is your sex drive?
10   Are you a stressful person?

Symptom Questionnaire

I have devised the following questionnaire to help you assess your symptoms and medical history. *Use this questionnaire only as a guide. It is essential you consult a qualified doctor or complementary practitioner before beginning any treatment or supplement programme.*

Self-assessment questionnaire

Complete each of the sections below and total your score at the end. Add each of the sections together and analyze your total score.

SECTION A: PAST HISTORY

POINTS AS FOLLOWS: 10 POINTS FOR EACH 'YES'

1. Is there a history of thyroid disease in your family?
YES / NO ....points

2. Have you at anytime required throat or neck surgery e.g. tonsillitis?
YES / NO ....points

3. Have you ever been the victim of a road traffic accident involving neck injury e.g. whip-lash injury?
YES / NO ....points

4. Have you in the past suffered from any of the following conditions: glandular fever, systemic candidiasis, hepatitis, chronic fatigue syndrome or anorexia nervosa?
YES / NO ....points

5. Have you a history of chronic constipation?
YES / NO   ....points

6. Have you a history of high blood pressure?
YES / NO   ....points

7. Have you a history of depression?
YES / NO   ....points

8. Have you ever been seriously overweight, e.g. 20% over optimal
weight?
YES / NO   ....points

9. Have you had a general anaesthetic in the previous two years?
YES / NO   ....points

10. If you have been pregnant, did any of the following health
problems occur? Miscarriage, obesity, post-partum (natal) depression
or thyroid imbalance.
YES / NO   ....points

Total for Section A ....points

SECTION B: CURRENT SYMPTOMS

POINTS AS FOLLOWS:

5 POINTS IF THE SYMPTOM IS TRIVIAL AND / OR OCCASIONAL

10 POINTS IF THE SYMPTOM IS MODERATE AND/OR FREQUENT

15 POINTS IF THE SYMPTOM IS SEVERE AND/OR CONSTANT

1. Physical fatigue ....points
2. Poor concentration ....points
3. Poor short-term memory ....points
4. Depression ....points
5. Cold extremities (e.g. hands and feet) ....points
6. Muscle pain and cramping ....points
7. Generally feel worse just after waking up. ....points
8. Low libido (sex drive) ....points
9. Moody and irritable ....points
10. Anxiety ....points
11. Symptoms worse with missed meals ....points
12. PMS ....points
13. Heavy periods ....points
14. Constipation ....points
15. Dry skin and/or hair loss ....points
16. Unexplained weight increase ....points
17. Frequent infections (e.g. throat or lung infections) ....points
18. Headaches ....points
19. Catarrhal/nasal congestion ....points
20. Dizziness, poor balance ....points

Total for Section B ....points

SECTION C: TESTS AND TREATMENT

POINTS AS FOLLOWS: 100 POINTS FOR EACH 'YES'

1. Have you had a thyroid hormone blood test over the previous two years with a free T₄ under 15pmol/L or a TSH over 4. 0mU/L?
YES / NO   ....points

2. Have you in the past needed thyroid surgery or radioactive iodine treatment for 'hyperthyroidism'?
YES / NO   ....points

3. Have blood tests shown you to have a raised cholesterol?
YES / NO   ....points

4. Is your morning temperature (see page 129) constantly below 97.5°F (36.4°C)?
YES / NO   ....points

Total for Section C ....points

ANALYSIS

When you have arrived at a grand total score by adding Sections A, B and C together you can assess the likelihood of you having mild hypothyroidism as follows:

SCORE	MILD HYPOTHYROIDISM DIAGNOSIS
600–800	Almost certain
400–600	Probable
200–400	Possible
0–200	Unlikely

Summary

As I have mentioned above this type of assessment should only be seen as a rough guide. However, those readers whose scores total over '500 points' would be advised to seek professional help from a sympathetic medical doctor or a complementary practitioner who is familiar with thyroid disease and treatment, they can then carry out more detailed analysis.

Strategy B: Taking Your Early Morning Temperature

Your normal body temperature or basal temperature measurement (BTM) has for over 100 years been recognized as a valuable indicator of thyroid activity. (This is why I frequently ask patients if they are a 'cold or warm' person.)

Doctors and practitioners have noted that patients with a sluggish thyroid have below normal temperatures. This is not too surprising as we know that the thyroid has a direct effect on our metabolic rate and the metabolism has a direct influence on the body temperature. A fever reflects an attempt by the body to increase the immune response by raising the temperature. Our metabolic rate increases when the temperature increases and decreases when the temperature falls.

In the 1940s an American doctor Broda Barnes pioneered a systematic method of thyroid diagnosis, based on this early morning temperature evidence. I recommend you try this test as it is a safe and easy way to assess your vulnerability to hypothyroidism[1].

This is what you need to do:

1   Place a thermometer under the arm immediately upon waking, and retain for 10 minutes before checking.
2   Try to do this at the same time each day.
3   Test for at least three consecutive days.
4   Do not talk or move until the test is completed.
5   Men can check the temperature on any three days. For women who are menstruating the temperature is best measured on day 2, 3 and 4 of their period. Before puberty and after menopause, any three days will suffice.

Some doctors request women to test for 28 days to obtain more accurate average temperatures. This can become rather tedious, and I do find that an average of three or four days readings provides sufficient diagnostic information.

> Barnes recognized several other conditions which can influence a person's BTM. These include: anorexia or fasting conditions; adrenal exhaustion or hypoadrenalism; pituitary gland deficiency; chronic long-term infections; post-viral fatigue and chronic fatigue syndrome; coming off the contraceptive pill.

Temperatures

The 'normal' under tongue temperature for a healthy person is 98.6°F or 37°C, the 'normal' BTM, however, is in the range 97.8 – 98.2° F or 36.6 – 36.8°C. I have found that temperatures as low as 95.6°F or 35. 4°C are not unusual in hypothyroid patients.

Dr Barnes held the rather simplistic view that a morning temperature below 97.8°F indicated hypothyroidism while a temperature above 98.2° F indicated hyperthyroidism. Although the BTM is not a definitive test, nor is it 100 per cent accurate, when it is used in conjunction with the other methods of diagnosis in this chapter it is a useful indicator of hypothyroidism and offers a valuable means to monitor progress under treatment. The temperature increase associated with improvement is often evident before there is any symptom relief, and before the levels of the thyroid blood tests show an improvement. It offers a subtle indication for thyroid change.

Although the Barnes Basal Temperature measurement is seen as the standard method to identify low temperatures, other methods are in use.

Dr E. Denis Wilson (author of Wilson's Syndrome) requests his patients to check their mouth temperatures three hours after waking and then again at six hours and nine hours. For example if they wake at 7.30am the temperatures are checked at 10.30am, 1.30pm and 4.30pm. Dr Wilson offers three reasons for preferring this type of testing:

1. Morning tests can give false positives as our temperature is normally low with sleeping. Therefore a day-time average offers more validity.

2. Temperatures can fluctuate quite quickly so an average of three readings over six hours is more reliable than a single reading.

3. Mouth temperatures are easier and faster to check than underarm measurements.

I share Dr Wilson's views on thermometers. He prefers the traditional glass thermometer and considers that the digital type thermometers can be unreliable[2].

Assessing Your Weight

I would also suggest you do this simple equation to assess your body mass index (BMI). This will give you a realistic view on whether you are over or underweight.

Your BMI is more accurate than simple scales as it takes into account your height (not, however, fat content or bone weight). Work it out as follows:

Your weight in kilograms divided by square of your height in metres.

Example: My height is 1.83m and my weight 76kg. My BMI is therefore $76 \div 1.83 \times 1.83$ or $76 \div 3.35 = 22.7$.

The ideal scale is as follows:

BMI

20–25	Normal weight
25–30	Overweight
30–40	Seriously overweight
40 +	Dangerously overweight

These various weights can be a little confusing, but they are a useful guide and are still employed by health practitioners to diagnose the metabolic rate and optimum weight of a hypothyroid patient.

Assessing Your Metabolic Rate

This is another traditional way of assessing thyroid disorders which was employed before laboratory testing was introduced. The assessment of a patient's **basal metabolic rate** (BMR) was one of the earliest tests used to detect hypothyroidism. However, it is not very accurate and the results are susceptible to change with different temperatures.

Nowadays practitioners test a patient's **resting metabolic rate** (RMR). This is expressed in calories and indicates the amount of liberated heat that occurs with the metabolic process. This sounds rather complicated but a simple self-assessment test can be done as follows:

* If you age is below 30 multiply your weight (in kilograms) by 14.7 and add 500.
* If your age is over 30, multiply your weight by 8.7 and add 830.

Remember that the RMR is your 'resting' calorific profile. Exercise, temperature changes, digestive efficiency and our hormone balance can all increase our calorific need by stepping up our metabolic rate. To arrive at an appropriate figure for your daily calorific intake you will therefore have to adjust the figure from the above sums.

1   If you have an active job and you do regular exercise multipy your RMR by 2.
2   If you have a sedentary job, but take a little daily exercise multiply your RMR by 1.7.
3   If you have a sedentary job and do no exercise multiply your RMR by 1.4.

Examples

* Jane: A 1.63m (5ft 4in.) woman of 25 years and weighing 50kg (112lb) who had a desk job and did little exercise would require 1,725 calories daily.
* Paul: A 1.95m (6ft 4in) man of 50 and weighing 87kg (196lb) who had an active job and cycled to and from work everyday would require 3,180 calories daily.

It is easy to see therefore how much difference exercise makes and how easily modern processed food can up calorie intake to above the daily recommended amount, causing weight to be put on.

Use this guide to work out your metabolic requirements. It is only a guide and as mentioned before the information should always be presented to a medical practitioner or complementary therapist. However, if you are overweight, yet feel you take in a healthy amount of calories, you may have a thyroid deficiency and I would recommend you see a professional about your concerns.

Strategy C: Laboratory Tests

Once you have completed the questions and tests above, the next step is to see a doctor or complementary health practitioner experienced in thyroid disorders. Even if some of the questions above do not seem appropriate, it is always necessary to talk to a health professional about *any* concerns you may have. A health practitioner will not only investigate many different lines of inquiry, but will also ease your mind and calm any fears. The information in this book is intended as a guide; you should use the information in this section to show your practitioner your symptoms in a clear and concise way, treatment must then be undertaken *under strict supervision*.

Now, once you do see a health practitioner they will undertake some or all or the laboratory tests below.

Hormone Testing

As I explained in chapter one (see pages 7–15) the thyroid gland release two hormones, thyroxine (T4) and triiodothyronine (T3). Separate blood tests are able to detect how much of each hormone is being released by the thyroid gland. Unfortunately, measuring the amount of thyroid hormones in the blood does not always reflect the functional efficiency of thyroid hormones in the cells.

Many doctors and researchers therefore see the blood measurement of another hormone, as the best guide to thyroid function. This is the thyroid stimulating hormone (TSH) or thyrotropin, and it is released from the anterior lobe of the pituitary gland which is situated beneath the brain. As you have seen from figure 1 on page 11 the pituitary itself is controlled by the hypothalamus in the brain which releases the hormone thyrotropin releasing hormone (TRH) to control the TSH status. This system works on a negative feedback system (see figure 1 page 11). The TSH and TRH being releases in response to low levels of T4. When the blood levels of T4 rise the TSH and TRH triggers are stopped.

Therefore the TSH level increases when the thyroid is underactive and decreases when the thyroid is overactive.

For the testing of mild hypothyroidism I usually obtain all the information that is required for the diagnosis and future monitoring by requesting a thyroid profile test consisting of a TSH and a free T4.

Free T4 is usually requested in preference to free T3. Essentially the free T3 is not so reliable or so useful as the free T4. This is partly because T3 can be released by a depressed thyroid gland more easily than T4. Therefore the level of T3 falls more slowly than T4 under conditions of hypothyroidism. Many non-thyroid illnesses also cause a reduction in the blood T3 without involving the thyroid. This is termed 'sick euthyroid' syndrome. Recovery from the non-thyroid illness usually returns the T3 status to normal.

Testing for T₃ and T₄ involves four blood tests. These being:

Total (protein-bound) T₃
Free T₃
Total (protein-bound) T₄
Free T₄

Total tests indicate that the T₃ or T₄ is bound to protein carriers. The chief drawback encountered when measuring total levels is the variable amount of protein bound to the hormones. More than 40 drugs, HRT, the contraceptive pill and pregnancy, can all cause variation in the carrier proteins leading to unreliable results.

This is why free T₃ and free T₄ are more frequently requested. The small amounts of free (unbound) T₃ and T₄ in the blood are the active constituents of the total hormones. They are therefore diagnostically more reliable and significant.

Cholesterol Testing

The link between blood cholesterol levels and thyroid function was first discussed in 1918[3]. It was observed that the blood cholesterol levels in animals decreased when they were given desiccated thyroid[4].

It was demonstrated in the 1930s that patients with hyperthyroidism showed low blood cholesterol (often well below the normal range). After surgery to remove part of the thyroid, the cholesterol level increased to above the normal, suggesting that too much thyroid tissue had been removed rendering the patient hypothyroid. If the patient was then given thyroid treatment, the cholesterol levels normalized.[5]

All this caused considerable excitement in the 1930s. Many researchers and doctors became convinced that if thyroid hormones controlled the blood cholesterol levels in many patients, measuring the cholesterol offered a very useful test to assess thyroid function.

Broda Barnes, however, found that, 'Blood cholesterol cannot be depended upon as a universal indicator of hypothyroidism'. His research confirmed that in young patients the cholesterol level can be normal regardless of thyroid activity, and even in elderly patients a correlation between low thyroid and high cholesterol could not always be demonstrated[6].

Protein Bound Iodine (PBI)

Around 100 years ago it was known that iodine was essential for thyroid function and that this trace element was bound to a large protein molecular carrier.

It was therefore assumed that measuring the iodine bound to protein in the blood, would provide a figure for the amount of circulating thyroid hormones. The test is called 'PBI' or 'protein bound iodine'. Unfortunately, extra iodine in a person's diet (from iodised salt, cough mixtures etc.) tends to combine with other proteins that are not carriers, leading to a masking of hypothyroidism by raising low values to within the normal range.

By the 1950s more thyroid hormone testing was developed and the PBI is now rarely requested.

Summary of Diagnosis

Diagnosis of mild hypothyroidism should, in my view, be based on the three factors outlined through the beginning of this chapter.

1   Assessment of history, signs and symptoms.
2   Taking your own body temperature (BTM).
3   Laboratory tests requested by a health practitioner.

Symptoms of hypothyroidism can be misleading, resulting in the frequent under-diagnosing of the condition. Unfortunately there exist many health problems that show very similar symptom patterns to hypothyroidism.

However, by combining these three strategies – the first two which you can conduct at home – you can thoroughly assess whether you may have hypothyroidism.

CHAPTER TEN

Treating Your Mild Hypothyroidism

Now that we have looked at the major symptoms of mild hypothyroidism and the methods of diagnosis, it is time to look at how you can overcome your fatigue and depression and restore your vitality. There are three main avenues for treating hypothyroidism:

A   Medical treatment
B   Naturopathic treatment
C   Recovery through diet

If your weight is of concern, eating the healthy Mediterranean diet discussed on pages 156–161 should be used in combination with one of the other medical or naturopathic treatments. However, even if your weight is normal, your hypothyroid symptoms can be greatly alleviated through diet. I would therefore recommend all readers diagnosed with hypothyroidism to follow the Mediterranean diet.

Strategy A: Medical Treatment

The standard medical treatment of mild hypothyroidism in the UK usually consists of a prescription for thyroxine (T₄) or in the US a combination of thyroxine and triiodothyronine (T₃). Unfortunately, as I have outlined in chapter one, mild or subclinical hypothyroidism is rarely diagnosed.

The excessively broad UK reference range for the free T₄ blood test usually ensures that only severely low levels are diagnosed and treated. The current tests requested to assess thyroid function are not considered sensitive enough to identify mild levels of underactivity. Furthermore, although the patient's symptoms can provide useful confirmation, these are often discounted, particularly if the test results are within the 'normal range'.

A few far-sighted UK doctors, (often in the private sector) prescribe whole animal thyroid. This is usually pig's thyroid and is sold as Armour.

You may already have been diagnosed as hypothyroid and therefore taking thyroid replacement treatment i.e. thyroxine. For this reason, and also for general interest, it is worthwhile answering the typical questions that I am frequently asked concerning thyroxine treatment.

'How is thyroxine made and what does it contain? Is it suitable for vegans and orthodox Jews?'

Thyroxine is synthetically 'man-made'. It is, however, chemically identical to our own natural hormone. No animal products are involved in its production, making it quite suitable for use by vegans, orthodox Jews and any other groups who are concerned with animal welfare or animal protein-free supplements and diets.

'What are the (tablet) strengths?'

Thyroxine is prescribed as a small tablet in strengths of 25, 50, 100 and 200 micrograms (mcg). A microgram is a thousandth of a milligram (mg), therefore 0.1mg is the same as 100mcg and 25mcg is also 0.025mg. The dimensions of thyroxine tablets are not standardized, and dosages are defined in milligrams or micrograms, so be on the alert to your exact prescription requirements.

Thyroxine is a stable substance with a long shelf life.

'What are typical doses?'

The usual dosage of thyroxine ranges from 25mcg to 200mcg. The average prescription being between 100mcg and150mcg. Many doctors will start treatment at 50mcgms and increase when indicated by 25mcg every two or three weeks, up to the patient's optimum dosage. Elderly patients with heart disorders, may need to start on 25mcg daily, as thyroxine can speed up the metabolism, including the heart.

Your appropriate dosage of thyroxine is determined by your response to treatment.

'How long do I take thyroxine?'

As thyroxine is prescribed as a replacement therapy, it is usually seen as a lifelong treatment. (This being similar to an insulin dependent diabetic.)

For this reason thyroxine and insulin are provided in many countries as free prescriptions. However, patients with very mild or short-term hypothyroidism, who are on a low dosage of thyroxine (e.g. 25mcg) have been known to successfully discontinue treatment after recovery.

'How quickly does it work?'

Thyroxine does not work very quickly. When a tablet is taken, there is unlikely to be any noticeable change to your metabolism for four or five days. Regarding long-term symptoms, it may take three to six months before blood improvement changes are noticed. As with many other disorders the duration of symptoms usually correlates with the recovery time; for example, if a patient has been fatigued and overweight as a result of an underactive thyroid for eight to 10 years, it may be nine to 12 months before full symptom recovery is achieved.

'How soon will my weight decrease?'

For many patients with thyroid deficiency, their excess weight is their chief concern. Unfortunately excess weight is very rarely the first symptom to improve. The overweight and the fatigue of hypothyroidism usually discourages exercise and sport. Although treatment may improve the mental and physical energy, it may be some months before the metabolic rate is successfully 'kick-started' leading to weight reduction. However, once the thyroid begins to normalize, any exercise and diet programme that is followed will become more successful.

'What are the side effects?'

Any side effects that result from thyroxine therapy usually fall into four groups.

1 Symptoms that arise when patients start the treatment.

Thyroxine stimulates the metabolism, and even young patients may experience quite harmless heart palpitations when treatment starts.

2　Symptoms that can develop with elderly patients.

Elderly patients have been known to develop symptoms of temporary heart malfunction when they begin to take thyroxine. These include rapid pulse (tachycardia), shortness of breath (dyspnoea), and even swollen ankles and angina with chest pain. Middle-aged and elderly patients with long-term thyroid deficiency may experience symptoms similar to muscular rheumatism. These include muscular aches and stiffness in the arms, legs and back. Many of the symptoms clear as treatment proceeds and a normal thyroid balance is gradually achieved.

3　Symptoms caused by patients taking too much thyroxine. This is often self-prescribed in the mistaken belief that they will lose weight more speedily.

Taking an inappropriate excess of thyroxine on a self-prescription basis can cause short-term heart symptoms and long-term bone calcium loss leading to osteoporosis.

4　Diabetic patients on insulin may experience episodes of hypoglycaemia if they become hypothyroid.

Insulin dependent diabetics may need to be particularly cautious when starting on thyroxine. Hypothyroidism can lower the blood sugar causing a diabetic patient to require less insulin. The opposite applies when the replacement thyroxine raises the thyroid output. This requires a careful balancing of insulin dosage requirements for the initial two to three months of thyroxine treatment. Patients who regularly use insulin and are experiencing unexplained and frequent 'hypos' (sudden falls in the blood sugar), are advised to request a thyroid test. This diabetes–hypothyroid link can easily be missed.

'Does thyroxine affect people differently e.g. young and old?'

There are no set rules regarding thyroxine dosage and age. Some patients require more thyroxine as they grow older and their thyroid becomes more deficient. However, many people require less thyroxine as they age.

This unpredictability and lack of a reliable pattern in age-related thyroxine dosages confirms the need for regular annual blood tests to monitor any changes.

'What if I become pregnant and/or breast feed?'

Patients with severe thyroid deficiency are unlikely to become pregnant. At one time it was routine to increase the thyroxine dose with pregnancy. This has been replaced now by frequent blood testing during pregnancy to observe any changes. Tests every three months are usually requested. If there is a need for an increase of thyroxine during pregnancy, the pre-pregnancy dosage can usually be returned to four to six weeks after childbirth.

The thyroid of the developing foetus is quite independent of the mother and produces its own hormones. Therefore breast feeding is quite safe when the mother is taking thyroxine.

'Does thyroxine combine beneficially with glandulars and other supplements?'

I regularly prescribe raw glandular thyroid supplements to patients who are taking thyroxine. This combination can be seen as an effective 'fine-tuning' of the thyroid. It can reduce the need for higher dosages of thyroxine, which can only increase the patient's dependency. It is also worth remembering that thyroxine or T_4 is only one of the hormones produced by the thyroid. The use of raw glandular thyroid ensures total thyroid support.

Strategy B: Naturopathy

As a naturopath specializing in thyroid and blood sugar disorders, this second approach to hypothyroid treatment is, in my experience, the most successful. As I have mentioned above, thyroxine only supplies one of the key hormones necessary for effective thyroid function, naturopathic treatment is far more comprehensive.

Naturopathy, as defined by the manifesto of the British Naturopathic Association, is 'A system of treatment which recognizes the existence of a vital curative force within the body'. Roger Newman Turner in his definitive book *Naturopathic Medicine* claims that 'The fundamental basis of naturopathy is the "vis medicatrix natural"' – the healing power of nature. He further states that 'Naturopathy is based on the recognition that the body possesses not only a natural ability to resist disease but inherent mechanisms of recovery and self-regulation'[1].

Clinically, naturopaths make use of hydrotherapy, dietetics and exercise. Many alternative or complementary therapies are usually seen to be under the naturopathic umbrella. These include herbalism, homoeopathy, acupuncture, osteopathy and chiropractic.

Unfortunately, very little research work or clinical trials have been carried out to prove that naturopathic concepts and methods actually work. You will appreciate that drug companies who usually finance medical research, would not be interested in funding trials into drug-free therapies. Although naturopathic methods are still vigorously employed in some of the German and Italian health hydros, the current trend in UK hydros has shown an emphasis for slimming and beauty therapies, indeed very sick patients are now rarely accepted at British hydros.

The naturopathic tenets may appear slightly old-fashioned and unscientific, but nutritional medicine is becoming increasingly recognized as a valuable component of modern medicine. Many naturopaths now use laboratory tests as an aid to diagnosis. The combination of functional health testing, coupled with traditional naturopathic treatment modalities, can offer safe and effective health care. One of my colleagues always responds to the question 'What is naturopathy?' by saying 'naturopaths treat people not diseases'. If you have been passed from one medical specialist to another medical specialist, without any relief from your symptoms, this answer can be very reassuring.

This naturopathy section outlines my own treatment approach for mild or low grade hypothyroidism. The chief symptom caused by this condition is undoubtably fatigue, but successful treatment can also resolve the many other diverse symptoms that are caused by an under-functioning thyroid gland.

Although specific thyroid support is usually required for each patient, other health problems and symptoms may also need to be treated. I do not have a standard treatment strategy for every patient with mild hypothyroidism. As the case histories in this book demonstrate, each patient is different and their supplement programmes and diets need to be designed with their individual requirements in mind.

Raw Glandular Therapy

Animal tissue concentrates also termed 'protomorphogens' or 'organ-specifics', have been in use for thousands of years. The like-cures-like basis of this therapy, rests on the assumption that by using animal glands the appropriate nutrient proportions can be provided as are found in our own organs and glands. The glandular preparations in current use are called raw because no heat is used in their processing. The glands are taken from Canadian corn fed cattle. After removal, the glands are de-fatted and kept frozen until processed. The critics of raw glandulars (or 'cow parts' as they have named them), argue that they fail to be clinically effective for two reasons.

1   The material contained in the glands is reduced to basic
    amino acids (the building blocks of protein) in the process of
    digestion, and therefore does not possess any specific thera-
    peutic value. The glandular detractors argue that the patients
    who take glandular supplements would obtain the same
    'benefits' by eating any type of protein (e.g. fish, meat, cheese
    or egg).
2   The other argument against tissue specifics in therapy claims
    that unless proteins are broken down into simple amino-acids
    they cannot be absorbed from the gut and passed into the
    bloodstream, as they would be too large.

There is evidence available to show that when enzymes and proteins
are eaten and absorbed through the gut lining, approximately 50 per
cent passes into the blood. Significantly this is in the form of molecules that have not been reduced to amino acids. Leon Chaitow
states in his book *The Raw Materials of Health*, 'Furthermore, and
of critical significance to the concept of using specific organs and
glands in therapy, it is known that at least 20 per cent of these
unchanged [by digestion] protein molecules retain their original
characteristics'[2].

It seems likely therefore that when raw glandular supplements
are properly prepared from healthy free-range animals, they provide
a specific therapeutic value for the gland that is targeted.

> The nutritional make-up of the glands and organs of
> animals are chemically very similar to their human
> counterparts. It follows, therefore, that the specific
> nutritional constituents which are provided by such a
> system will be in the optimum ratios and quantities.

The Results of Glandular Therapy Use

When patients are prescribed thyroxine for their underactive thyroid, subsequent blood tests usually show that their blood thyroxine (free T4) has increased. This is not too surprising as the increase simply reflects their daily dose of thyroxine. Unfortunately the improvement in the blood is not always paralleled by symptom improvement. Furthermore taking thyroxine does not guarantee an increase in the efficiency of their thyroid. In fact by artificially introducing a hormone, the gland concerned can become less efficient, thus reducing its output. For this reason the prescription for thyroxine in the UK is a free prescription as a dependency is created and the prescribed thyroxine is required until the patient dies.

With the use of thyroid tissue supplements, however, the blood thyroxine improves as a direct result of the patient's thyroid becoming more efficient. When this improvement leads to symptom relief, and the blood test results improve, the thyroid tissue can be discontinued or continued on a low maintenance dosage. The latter usually applies to very elderly patients or patients who have experienced symptoms for many years.

Dosages and Maintenance

The list below of patients who have benefited from raw glandular therapy indicates the changes in their blood T4, over various periods of time.

Free T₄ Changes in Patients Taking 'T-Lyph'

DOSAGE: 6 tablets daily (totalling 780mg raw glandular thyroid of bovine source).

PATIENT	AGE	PERIOD	FREE T^4
Miss W	41		12.4pmol/L
		12 months	14.1pmol/L
Mrs S	39		10.1pmol/L
		4 months	12.6pmol/L
Mrs Z	45		11.6pmol/L
		3 months	13.4pmol/L
Miss K	49		9.9pmol/L
		7 months	11.2pmol/L
		9 months	15.7pmol/L
Mrs R	52		12.5pmol/L
		12 months	19.7pmol/L
Mrs P	68		11.7pmol/L
		3 months	17.0pmol/L
Mrs T	55		7.7pmol/L
		3 months	13.5pmol/L
		5 months	14.4pmol/L
Mrs J	52		10.7pmol/L
		3 months	12.2pmol/L
		6 months	13.0pmol/L

Mr W	56		10.6pmol/L
		3 months	12.6pmol/L
Mrs C	29		10.2pmol/L
		6 months	14.3pmol/L

The thyroid is a notoriously slow gland to respond to any treatment and for this reason many physicians only request a blood test every six or 12 months. However, I do find that a three-monthly blood test review can be worthwhile, to identify progress.

Unfortunately there is not a generally accepted standard level of free T_4 that guarantees symptom relief. As you will be aware from chapter 1, there is a great variation in the size and function of the thyroid gland. For this reason I usually request a blood test when patients feel symptom-free and have a satisfactory level of energy. Such a result serves as a useful guide for the rest of their lives, as it reflects their 'normal' level of blood thyroxine. Any return of symptoms in the future need only be assessed by further blood thyroid tests, which can then be compared with their established norm.

Non-Glandular Supplements

There is currently only one company in the UK that markets thyroid glandular supplements. The supplements are named T-Lyph and T-Lyph Three. These are available from Nutri Ltd (see suppliers page 234) who only supply direct to the practitioner or direct to the patient with a practitioner's order.

Nutri Ltd also markets Core Level Thyro which is a 'synergistic thyroid support' providing vitamins, minerals, amino acids and herbs as a general thyroid support. However, I have recently formulated a non-glandular thyroid support for Nutri Ltd named Thyro-Complex™. The constituents of which include all the precursors of thyroxine and the nutrients required to facilitate the effective conversion of T$_4$ to T$_3$ In addition, the vitamins, minerals, amino acids and herbs known to be essential for effective thyroid metabolism.

Constituents of Thyro-Complex™

Amounts refer to two tablets

L-Tyrosine	500mg
L-Carnitine	250mg
DL-Phenylalanine	250mg
Iodine (kelp)	150mcg
Licorice Root	20mg
Vitamin A (palmitate)	1500mcgm
Folic Acid	150mcgs
Vitamin B1 (thiamine HC1)	10mg
Vitamin B2 (riboflavin)	10mg
Vitamin B3 (niacin)	25mg
Vitamin B6 (pyridoxineHC1)	25mg
Vitamin C	500mg
Vitamin E	200IU
Selenium (aspartate)	50mcg
Zinc (picolinate)	8mg
Calcium (aspartate)	80mg
Magnesium (aspartate)	50mg
Copper (chelate)	1mg
Manganese (chelate)	3mg

I have known patients who have refused to take thyroid glandulars on religious and nutritional grounds (these include vegans and orthodox Jews). Although the Thyro-Complex™ was designed to back up the glandular treatment, it also provides an efficient non-glandular thyroid boost for those patients who choose not to take animal products.

Strategy C: Diets for Hypothyroidism

Unlike many other ailments, I do not know of a universally accepted standard diet that is recommended for hypothyroidism. However, the symptoms and health conditions that develop as a result of low thyroid function provides clues to the appropriate dietary requirements.

I believe that these symptoms can be greatly alleviated through diet, and for those of you who may have excess weight, this diet can help you to lose it safely and slowly.

Weight Loss and Hypothyroidism

In western nations the incidence of female obesity is around 40 per cent. Millions of pounds are spent annually on diet books, magazines, special foods and drinks and dieting clubs and support groups. I believe that reducing calories to lose weight can only work on two provisions:

REGULAR EXERCISE

1   Exercise during and after weight loss needs to be considered and slotted into the dieter's lifestyle. Examples of the calories required for exercise are as follows:

Exercise for one hour	Calories consumed
Walking (slowly)	200 cal
Bowling	200 cal
Dancing	300 cal
Gardening	300 cal
Walking (fast)	300 cal
Cycling	600 cal
Playing golf (two hours)	600 cal

Swimming	600 cal
Jogging	600 cal
Playing football	600 cal

STABLE METABOLISM

2   Your metabolism has been stabilized and any thyroid disorder diagnosed and treated.

Research has shown that the metabolic rate can be increased by over 25 per cent for up to 15 hours after strenuous exercise such as running or swimming.

Significantly, the rate can still be increased by 10 per cent for as long as 48 hours after exercise. This indicates that daily exercise is not absolutely essential, and dieters can plan an exercise regime for every other day with good results. Although, as can be seen, exercise reduces calories, it also serves to maintain the metabolic rate during the diet and after the dieting and weight loss is over.

THE GLYCAEMIC INDEX

It is not only important to follow a low fat diet when pursuing a healthy eating regime, but also to follow a low sugar diet. The glycaemic index ranks foods according to the rise in the blood sugar (glucose) after consumption. The higher the increase in the blood sugar after eating a particular food, the higher the food will be in the index. Not surprisingly sugars and refined carbohydrates have a high glycaemic index factor, and complex carbohydrates, fats and proteins (brown pasta and vegetables etc.) have a lower factor. The most rapidly absorbed food is glucose itself – which has been given the arbitrary GI number of 100.

The list below taken from my book *Diets to Help Migraine* includes some common foods with their glycaemic index numbers[3]. As a general guideline foods with a GI less than 50 can be seen as low GI and foods over 50 are termed medium to high GI.

The Glycaemic Index

Sugars	GI
Glucose	100
Honey	87
Sucrose	59
Fructose	20

Cereals	
Cornflakes	80
Wholegrain bread	72
White rice	72
White bread	69
Brown rice	68
Shredded Wheat	67
Swiss muesli	66
Sweetcorn	59
All Bran	51
Spaghetti	50
Oatmeal cereal	49
Wholewheat spaghetti	42

Fruit	
Raisins	64
Banana	62
Orange juice	46
Apple juice	45
Orange	40
Apple	39

Vegetables

Parsnip	97
Carrot	92
Mashed potato	80
Potato	70
Beetroot	64
Frozen peas	51
Peas	33

Pulses

Baked beans	40
Lima beans	36
Kidney beans	29
Lentils	29
Soya beans	15

Dairy Products

Yoghurt (plain)	36
Ice-cream	36
Whole milk	34
Skimmed milk	32

Various

Chocolate bar	68–75
Potato chips	51
Sponge cake	46
Digestive biscuits	45
Peanuts	13

Here are some specific diet recommendations for treating some of the most common symptoms of hypothyroidism (these we covered in Part One).

FATIGUE
Low sugar diet with plenty of low GI foods and avoiding high GI foods. Iron rich foods may also be required. Protein food should be part of each meal to reduce insulin resistance and any tendency to low blood sugar.

> Insulin resistance: This term defines the effects of the typical high sugar–refined carbohydrate western diet. The high blood sugar leads to an overproduction of insulin (hyperinsulinism) and a resulting stimulation of fat storage. In times of food shortage, to be able to produce an excess of insulin encouraged a useful storage capability as the excess blood glucose was converted into fat. Unfortunately, in the high calorie-food excess 20th century, our metabolism has not adjusted to the overabundance of food and so our surplus calories are still stored as fat. Unless we exercise regularly, our body fat and blood fats can increase causing a variety of health problems.

CARDIOVASCULAR SYMPTOMS
Low fat and low sugar diet, avoiding tobacco.
Increase of foods rich in omega 3 EFAs (e.g. fish and various oils)

IMMUNE SYSTEM WEAKNESS
Foods rich in antioxidants (see page 204)

ANAEMIA
Iron rich foods

SKIN SYMPTOMS
Low sugar, low animal fat diet, rich in foods containing omega 3, EFAs, zinc and beta carotene (vitamin A).

GOITREGENS
It is generally wise to avoid excesses of the goitregen rich foods (see page 206).

The Ideal Diet for Treating Hypothyroidism

As you will begin to understand after reading the above guidelines, there are several key elements that constitute an ideal diet for hypothyroidism. I believe many of these elements can be found in the diet of the Eastern Mediterranean. Although the towns and cities are gradually changing to a high fat, high sugar convenience foods regime, the rural diets of Southern France, Italy, Greece and the Greek Islands still include some of the healthiest foods in the world. The low incidence of heart disease, obesity, diabetes and other diseases speaks for itself.

According to the World Health Organization's Statistical Annual for 1989, the incidence of fatal heart attacks in America is roughly twice that of Italy and Greece. In America well over one million people die from cardiovascular disease each year.

The term 'Mediterranean Triad' was first coined by Paul Mac-Kendrick[4] to describe the three key elements of the regional diets of Greece, Italy and Southern France. This triad consists of wheat, olives and grapes. The climate of the Mediterranean region – which includes hot dry summers and mild rainy winters – provides ideal conditions for growing durum wheat, olive trees and vines. The deep roots of the olive trees and vines protects them from the summer drought, and the short growing period of the durum wheat harvest, ensures a crop before the summer heat. In the past, the shortage of water meant that crops traditionally needed to be processed and stored to last throughout the year, without refrigeration. Wheat can be processed into flour, pasta or semolina. Olives are easily preserved and olive oil can be kept almost indefinitely. Grapes can be eaten fresh, dried (currants and raisins) or made into wine. In addition to the three staples, fish, fowl, game, goats' cheese and yoghurt, vegetables, salads, garlic and onions and seasonal fruit are all part of the diet.

Sheep and goats are the traditional animals for eating in the area. However, they are usually worth more alive than dead, as they provide milk, cheese and wool. Even today many Mediterranean farmers only eat red meat once or twice a year. The aim of the diet is to eat whole grain products and fresh vegetables and fruit. It is important to reduce the total fat and sugar intake, while substituting olive oil and other oils for solid fats. I enclose a copy of one of my typical diet sheets that I provide for patients.

The Mediterranean Diet – Guidelines

Cooking vegetables

* Many vegetables are eaten raw in salads.
* Most vegetable dishes are variations on vegetable stews e.g. ratatouille. The foundation of these stews being garlic and onion fried in olive oil.
* To conserve flavour and nutrient value, cook fresh vegetables in very little water or steam.
* A pressure cooker or microwave is ideal – do NOT add sugar or salt to any cooking vegetables.
* If unable to use fresh vegetables, frozen may occasionally be substituted.

* Canned vegetables usually contain a great deal of salt and their texture is poor.

Cooking with meat

* Meat from the Mediterranean area is naturally lean as there are few lush areas available. The Mediterranean countries do not go in for intensive factory farming which causes livestock to convert cereal to saturated fat.
* Mediterranean people eat very small amounts of meat in comparison to the entire meal.
* Red meat (veal and lamb) should only be eaten twice a week and white meat should have all skin and visible fat removed.

Cooking with fish

* The traditional Mediterranean methods of cooking fish includes grilling over charcoal (after brushing with olive oil), poaching (usually in wine), baking, and boiling (as in fish soup). For modern cooks, microwave cooking conserves flavours and food quality. On a critical note, the Mediterranean salt-cured fish is best avoided.
* Olive oil is ideal for the occasional frying. It can also be re-used if it has not been overheated. It should, however, be strained between use and if used to fry fish do not re-use with any other food.

Cooking with wine

* Wine can enhance the flavour of food. Either prepare a wine-enriched sauce for a meat, fish or chicken dish, or braise ingredients in a mixture of bouillion and wine for an hour or more.
* Some cuts of meat and fish can be marinated in wine. There is no alcohol content in the food as this is cooked away.

Dairy products

*   Low fat milk and dairy products are vital. Low fat spreads based on olive oil are now available in supermarkets.
*   Some continental cheeses contain less saturated fats than others e.g. feta, mozzarella and camembert. These cheeses can be included in any course or meal on the menu.
*   Plain low fat yoghurt is delicious, especially when used with fresh fruit for dessert.

Fresh fruit

*   A large bowl of seasonal fresh fruit should be available to end a meal, or to provide a healthy snack.

Olive oil

*   Today there are many varieties of olive oil available. It is recommended that you buy a small quantity of oil to begin with. Oils labelled 'virgin' vary in colour and flavour. Different grades of olive oil are used in salad dressings, to sauté, for deep frying and casseroles. Experimentation for personal taste – rather than recommendation – is the best answer.
*   Look for products packed in olive oil (tuna, artichoke hearts, sardines etc.).
*   *Extra Virgin Olive Oil*
*   Best quality oil from first pressing, giving a natural flavour.
*   *Virgin Olive Oil*
*   Slightly more piquant flavour.
*   *Olive Oil*
*   Blend of refined olive oil with extra virgin oil, making a quality oil suitable for all cooking purposes.

THE MEDITERRANEAN DIET

Breakfast

Fresh fruit juice, preferably freshly extracted and without sugar. Choose from:

a High fibre wholemeal cereal (without added sugar) with skimmed milk.
b Wholemeal or grain toast with peanut butter or olive oil spread, a little organic honey.
c Wholemeal or grain toast with scrambled, poached or boiled egg.
d Wholemeal or grain toast with sugar-free baked beans.
e A small omelette or sardines (in olive oil) on toast.
f A sliced peach or apricot (fresh or tinned in natural juice) with low fat natural yoghurt.
g Cup of herb tea or decaffeinated coffee with skimmed milk.

Lunch

The ideal is a raw salad with a selection from the following ingredients:

a Tomato, cucumber, raw cabbage, onion, garlic, green pepper, sardines, herring, tuna (in olive oil), olives, anchovies, young beetroot greens, coleslaw (cabbage and carrots), artichokes, stuffed vine leaves, thin slices of mozzarella cheese, hard-boiled eggs, cold new potatoes and spinach.
b Use olive oil and vinegar dressing (red or white wine).
c Drink one glass of dry white or red wine, or mineral water.

Dinner

Appetizers

a Hors d'oeuvres (selection of fresh vegetables and salad, served simply, avoid paté and sausage).
b Use olive oil/vinegar dressing.
c Antipasto, a selection of lean raw or cooked ham served with marinated vegetables.
d Small 'country-style' salad e.g. Salade Nicoise.
e Artichoke or asparagus vinaigrette.
f Stuffed vegetables served hot or cold (e.g tomato, courgette, aubergine [egg plant]).

Soups

a Lighter soups for summer e.g. gazpacho, borscht, garlic.
b Fish soup with aeoli (garlic mayonnaise).
c Soups for winter should be more substantial and contain pasta, rice or beans.
  e.g. minestrone, lentil.
d Good quality fresh seasonal 'home-made' soups can be obtained from supermarkets.

Main Meal

a Paella marinara
b Escalopes of veal and pasta
c Moussaka (Using minced veal or lamb.)
d Risotto
e Chicken dishes (All skin should be removed 'before' cooking.)
f Salad Nicoise
g Fish (Whole fish should be grilled having been brushed with olive oil first.)

h   Fillets can be poached, usually in wine.
i   Baked fish (Should be wrapped in paper/foil and cooked with various ingredients.)
j   Seafood salad

Dessert

a   Selection of seasonal fresh fruit
b   Cheese, including camembert, feta, mozzarella or goats' cheese – with or without wholegrain high-fibre crispbread etc.
c   Low fat natural yoghurt

Drink

a   One glass of dry white or red wine or mineral water
b   Cup of herb tea or decaffeinated coffee with skimmed milk

CHAPTER ELEVEN

Diagnosing the Causes of Fatigue

We are all different. Structurally, biochemically and emotionally we are unique. Although I have covered the diagnosis of hypothyroidism in chapter nine, the diagnosis of fatigue is altogether more complex. Fatigue is a symptom of many illnesses, yet to unravel any problem there must be a starting point. With this in mind I usually request laboratory tests and other tests on the basis of test>interpret results>discount or diagnose>treatment.

This means that a test is requested (an example being haemoglobin to diagnose an iron deficient anaemia). The results are then assessed in terms of the patient's signs and symptoms, diet, health history etc. and either eliminated from the diagnosis if negative or treated if the diagnosis is judged positive.

This type of sequence approach to testing ensures specificity in terms of diagnosis, at minimal cost for the patient. Having mentioned the price of medical testing I must add that I do not allow cost to compromise diagnostic accuracy. (Some physicians have been known to request tests with a research priority and not a patient's priority).

Very few patients require all the tests shown, and readers may be surprised at the variety and complexity of the tests that are available.

The procedure falls into three groups of tests. Should the results of group one prove to be inconclusive or negative, I then request group two, and finally if necessary group three if more evidence is needed for a satisfactory diagnosis. If, after group three, I have not obtained any conclusive or useful diagnostic clues I usually seek a second opinion. The procedure for interpreting test results varies with each physician, so a colleague's opinion can be useful. My protocol for test requesting with chronic fatigue is as follows:

Group One

Biochemistry Profile

This includes tests for kidney function, liver and gall bladder function, muscle damage, (including heart muscle), protein status, gout and blood sugar (for diabetes).

Lipid Profile (Fats)

This includes tests for total cholesterol, HDL and LDL cholesterol, the LDL-Total cholesterol ratio and the triglycerides.

Haematology Profile with Iron

This profile includes haemoglobin, red cells, white cells, platelets and the ESR (erythrocyte sedimentation rate).

Haemoglobin reflects the body's iron status as the red cell haemoglobin comprises up to 65 per cent of the total body iron. The remainder is contained in iron-containing enzymes (5 per cent), or stored as ferritin and haemosiderin (30 per cent). Iron stores can also be measured in the blood.

The platelets are involved in blood coagulation and high levels can lead to raised blood viscosity and clotting.

The ESR is raised in the presence of inflammation and infections.

There are various types of white cells that can be measured. The test is known as the differential white cell count. Examination of the white cells can provide clues to a wide range of diseases and imbalances.

Thyroid Profile

This is my most commonly requested test and includes Free T_3, Free T_4 and TSH.

To summarize group one. With a single syringe of blood 35 tests can be requested. This supplies valuable information on serious organ failure, anaemia, hypothyroidism, diabetes, gout, arthritis, immune deficiency and many other health problems. You will notice that nearly all these conditions feature fatigue as a major symptom.

If the results of the group one tests are normal or inconclusive I request all or some of the tests included in group two. These are largely tests for functional assessment, and tests to identify nutrient deficiencies.

GROUP TWO

Gut Permeability Profile

This requires the patient to take a small drink containing poly-ethylene glycol (PEG), a substance which cannot be absorbed, but passes out directly to the bladder. The PEG includes 11 different sized molecules and the normal recovery range is known for each molecule. The patient measures the urine passed over six hours following the drink, and a small sample of the urine with the fig-ure for the total amount passed is sent to the laboratory.

The elegant and very simple test which the patient does at home serves to identify a leaky gut or malabsorption. The three results below (A: leaky gut), (B: malabsorption), (C: normal), show typical graphs of three patients.

Serum and Red Cell Minerals

This blood test measures calcium, chromium, copper, iron, mag-nesium, manganese and zinc in the blood, and also the magne-sium in the red cells.

Red cell magnesium is seen as a valuable test for chronic fatigue patients, who often show a low level of magnesium.

Essential Fatty Acids in Red Blood Cells

This valuable test identifies the levels of the omega-3 and -6 series with other fatty acids (see page 213 for more information on EFAs).

A: Leaky Gut — Recovery in urine (6 hour collection)

Fraction	Molecular weight	Dose (Mg)	Mg	%	Reference range
1	198	4.0	1.4	**35.9**	26.6 – 33.4
2	242	9.0	3.2	**35.7**	26.5 – 31.6
3	286	39.0	13.3	**34.1**	25.2 – 29.4
4	330	96.0	28.2	**29.4**	21.1 – 25.0
5	374	157.0	41.6	**26.5**	17.9 – 22.0
6	418	171.0	32.7	**19.1**	12.5 – 16.2
7	462	176.0	22.2	**12.6**	6.4 – 10.8
8	506	145.0	14.1	**9.7**	3.6 – 6.0
9	550	105.0	6.3	**6.0**	1.0 – 2.4
10	594	67.0	1.6	**2.4**	Up to 1.4
11	638	31.0	0.4	**1.2**	Up to 0.7
	TOTAL:	1000.0	165.0	**16.5**	10.0 – 13.3%

Comments:

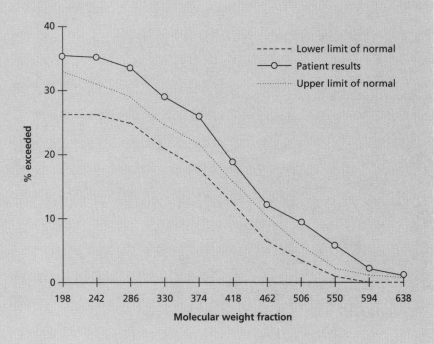

B: Malabsorption

Fraction	Molecular weight	Dose (Mg)	Recovery in urine (6 hour collection)		
			Mg	%	Reference range
1	198	4.0	1.0	24.9	26.6 – 33.4
2	242	9.0	2.2	24.1	26.5 – 31.6
3	286	39.0	9.0	23.2	25.2 – 29.4
4	330	96.0	15.4	16.0	21.1 – 25.0
5	374	157.0	14.8	9.4	17.9 – 22.0
6	418	171.0	8.2	4.8	12.5 – 16.2
7	462	176.0	3.9	2.2	6.4 – 10.8
8	506	145.0	1.5	1.0	3.6 – 6.0
9	550	105.0	0.4	0.4	1.0 – 2.4
10	594	67.0	0.0	0.0	Up to 1.4
11	638	31.0	0.0	0.0	Up to 0.7
	TOTAL:	1000.0	56.3	5.6	10.0 – 13.3%

Comments:

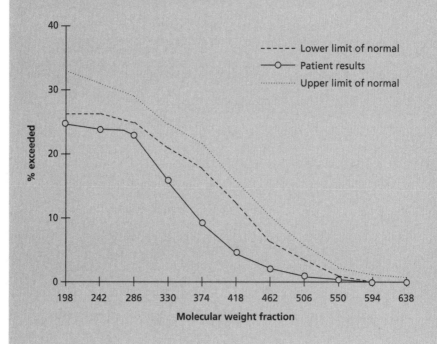

C: Normal			Recovery in urine (6 hour collection)		
Fraction	Molecular weight	Dose (Mg)	Mg	%	Reference range
1	198	4.0	1.1	28.2	26.6 – 33.4
2	242	9.0	2.5	28.2	26.5 – 31.6
3	286	39.0	10.5	27.0	25.2 – 29.4
4	330	96.0	22.3	23.2	21.1 – 25.0
5	374	157.0	32.0	20.4	17.9 – 22.0
6	418	171.0	25.1	14.7	12.5 – 16.2
7	462	176.0	14.4	8.2	6.4 – 10.8
8	506	145.0	5.8	4.0	3.6 – 6.0
9	550	105.0	1.1	1.0	1.0 – 2.4
10	594	67.0	0.2	0.3	Up to 1.4
11	638	31.0	0.0	0.0	Up to 0.7
	TOTAL:	1000.0	115.1	11.5	10.0 – 13.3%

Comments:

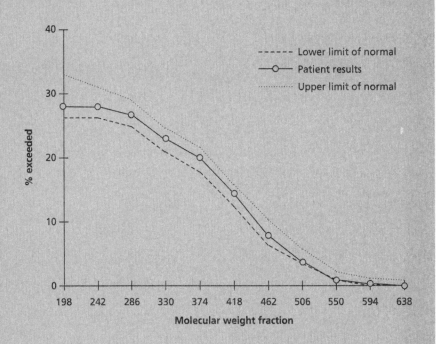

24-Hour Urine Amino Acid Test

This measures three groups of amino acids in the urine and includes a total of 38 amino acids.

Hair Mineral Analysis

This test is of special value when a toxic metal excess is suspected. Unlike the blood test for minerals, the hair analysis shows minerals stored in muscle, fat and liver tissue including the toxic minerals. These include lead, cadmium, mercury, arsenic and aluminium.

Haematinic Profile

This test provides a more detailed evaluation of the various types of anaemias. The test includes the measurement of iron, TIBC (total iron binding capacity) ferritin, serum vitamin B_{12}, and red cell folate (folic acid).

6-Hour Glucose Tolerance Test

The GTT is used to identify functional hypoglycaemia. A great deal of valuable information can be provided from the correct interpretation of the results. I believe, however, that it is essential to standardize the preparation for the test, the amount of glucose used and the timing of the sample taking.

Glucose Meters

Modern glucometers have a measuring range for blood glucose from 1.1mmol/L to 30+mmol/L. This makes them suitable for use in a seven sample GTT, particularly when testing very young and very old patients. I have, however, found that some meters tend to show a false reading with the blood droplet, when the finger is squeezed. Such pressure can cause tissue fluid to dilute the blood. However, the latest meters require a very small amount of blood, making excessive pressing and squeezing unnecessary.

Some UK labs give their patients a sugar flavoured drink which provides a non-standard sugar load. The American method of testing with 100gms of glucose I believe provides an excessive sugar surge in the blood, with a subsequently artificial response. I have always recommended 50gm of glucose, dissolved into two glasses of water with ¼ pint (150mls) in each glass. I request the patient to drink all the water within two minutes. Experience has shown me that if a patient is left alone in the rest room, they can sometimes take 20 minutes to drink the glucose solution. In recent years I have for this reason insisted on the time allowance, and the practice nurse ensures that this is followed.

GROUP 3

This group includes tests that look more closely at digestive efficiency, adrenal function, food intolerances, candidiasis, vitamin
deficiencies and intestinal parasites.

The tests include:

Candida Intensive Culture

This measures candida immune reactivity in the faeces and blood,
and provides a comprehensive profile.

Gastrogram

The patient needs to attend the laboratory for this gastric function test. A small capsule is swallowed and signals from the elec-
trodes contained in the capsule provide information on stomach
acidity (pH), stomach emptying speed and pancreatic enzyme levels. The test does not cause any discomfort to the patient, and
takes approximately 45 minutes. The capsule is passed and does
not need to be recovered.

Heliobacter Pylori Antibody

The heliobacter is seen as the main cause of gastric or stomach
ulcers in addition to being a risk factor for gastric cancer. This
simple blood test identifies its presence.

Although the antibody test is seen as a valuable screening tool, it
does not necessarily reflect current heliobacter activity or disease.
A more sophisticated test is the heliobacter urea breath test. This is
carried out at the laboratory, and is of particular value to ensure that
the anti-H pylori drug therapy has been successful.

Adrenal Stress Index or Profile

This valuable test involves measuring the DHEA and cortisol levels in four saliva samples taken over a 24-hour period.

DHEA-S

Dehydro-epiandrosterone sulphate is a blood test that is usually requested to monitor the effects of DHEA treatment. The sulphate form is secreated by the adrenal glands whilst DHEA is produced by the ovaries, the testes **and** the adrenals.

DHEA is converted in the body to the sulphate form, hence the value of the DHEA-S test.

Many doctors and naturopaths see this test as a useful indicator of the adrenal status, with adrenal exhaustion and general fatigue resulting from stress, the blood DHEA-S is often low.

Food Intolerance ELISA Test

The full name of this test is the 'Enzyme Linked Immunosorbent Assay'; this identifies the foods that the patient's immune system is reacting against. It can be assumed that if the blood develops immune complexes (IgG's) in response to specific, normally harmless foods, then the blood sees the food as a toxin.

Some confusion exists regarding the terms *allergy, sensitivity* and *intolerance*. I prefer the word intolerance when dealing with IgG reactions and consider allergies are more likely to be IgE reactions (as in peanuts, wasp stings etc.). There are five classes of immunoglobulins – IgA, IgD, IgE, IgG, and IgM. They are all antibodies present in the blood and other tissues which defend the body against various allergens. An allergen is the trigger that initiates a patient's allergic response, examples being food, dust, animal hair.

Various levels of intolerance are identified with the ELISA test and the specific foods must be either avoided or rotated. Many foods can be eaten freely. I find the avoidance of suspect foods for 6–8 weeks followed by the use of homoeopathic desensitising pillules and food rotation, usually allows a patient eventually to eat the suspected foods without symptoms developing.

Vitamin Measurements

Although the tests are costly, I sometimes request tests for blood vitamin levels. These include functional vitamin B_1 (thiamine) B_2 (riboflavin) and B_6 (pyridoxine), vitamin A, vitamin E and vitamin C.

In addition to requesting laboratory tests, a full case history is taken with each patient. This includes details on diet, exercise, lifestyle, employment, relationships, past health history and treatment. Weight, blood pressure, sleep patterns, family history and current stresses are also noted.

Comprehensive Digestive Stool Analysis with Parasitology

Parasitic and bacterial infection of the intestine are increasing throughout the world. The symptoms include the following:

Abdominal pain and cramp
Chronic fatigue
Diarrhoea
Distention and gastritis
IBS
Low back pain
Weight loss
Arthritis

Food intolerances
Crohn's disease
Malabsorption
Headache
Gut dysbiosis

This detailed stool analysis provides information on digestive efficiency and absorption, bacterial balance, parasites, yeast overgrowth, inflammation and immune function. Chronic gut imbalance can contribute to a range of health problems.

Summary

The groups listed above are requested to assist diagnosis and to identify the causes of chronic fatigue. Fatigue features as a major symptom of many diseases and the severity of the symptoms of coronary heart disease, cancer, kidney failure and chronic liver and lung disease serves to confirm the cause of the fatigue, and does not usually present problems with diagnosis. The majority of the chronically fatigued patients who consult me have not been diagnosed, they have usually been classed as clinically depressed, or their fatigue has been attributed to overwork, stress or the age factor.

Many of the tests that I have described, are not standard hospital tests and are therefore rarely requested by the patient's GP. It is logical to assume that there must be a reason when a person becomes exhausted. The object of testing for deficiencies, imbalances and malfunctions is to find the reasons why.

The psychologist William James stated that there could not be emotion without a physical change. Stress may often be caused by the way we think, but our ability to deal with, and survive stress, depends on the health of our endocrine system.

I am only tempted to tell a patient that their exhaustion is 'all in the mind' when the diagnostic procedures outlined above are unsuccessful.

The Causes of Mild Hypothyroidism

I believe there are many subtle and often missed causes of mild or low grade hypothyroidism. Many of these do not feature in the 'official' medical list of causes.

The early stages of diseases or abnormalities are termed 'subclinical'. This description is defined as 'before being detectable by clinical examination or laboratory tests'. Detection in this circumstance is dependent upon assessment of blood test results in the context of normal ranges. Many of the patients who consult me show symptoms that fit the possible diagnosis of mild hypothyroidism, however, they have usually been informed that their thyroid function tests are within the normal ranges, and that their thyroid must be working well; treatment is therefore not given.

Many doctors are very cautious when diagnosing hypothyroidism, chiefly because in medicine hypothyroidism is seen to describe a thyroid that is failing, and therefore requiring replacement hormone support. To justify such a prescription, biochemical evidence of an abnormal blood test finding is mandatory. This evidence usually consists of blood hormone results that are outside the normal ranges. The concept of a mildly underactive thyroid, causing symptoms but showing blood readings within the normal ranges is not generally accepted by medical doctors. The view that a gland can simply be inefficient or exhausted without being damaged or diseased, is also rarely acknowledged in medical diagnosis. Even when mild hypothyroidism is recognised it is not usually treated.

When hypothyroidism is diagnosed as a mildly functional, mainly reversible condition, an entirely different awareness of potential causes is called for. The major medical causes remain as suspects, but in addition many previously unsuspected factors need to be considered and treated, and where possible removed before the thyroid normalizes and good health is achieved.

Mainstream medical thinking identifies the following causes of hypothyroidism. These causes fall into eight main groups:

1) Congenital

Born without a thyroid (cretinism) or with an abnormal metabolic defect of the thyroid.

2) Inflammation of the Thyroid

As a result of a virus infection or Hashimoto's (Autoimmune syndrome).

3) Result of Previous Treatment

The treatment of hyperthyroidism can include surgical removal of part of the gland or the use of radioactive iodine. The iodine passes to the gland and being radioactive it causes destruction of thyroid tissue. Unfortunately both procedures can lead to a subsequent deficiency of the thyroid output, necessitating thyroxine replacement. Statistically, 70 per cent of such patients require thyroxine for 10 to

20 years after treatment for hyperthyroidism as their thyroid has passed from overactivity to underactivity.

4) Drugs

Many drugs reduce the level of, or inhibit the activity of, the thyroid hormones. They can also compromise the accuracy of blood test results. Examples are:

> Lithium (Priadel) – for psychiatric illness
> Phenylbutazone (Butacote) – for ankylosing spondylitis
> Tolbutamide (Rastinon) – used for treating diabetes
> Beta-blockers (Inderal) – for high blood pressure
> Salicylates (Disprin etc.) – analgesics
> Androgens (e.g. testosterone) – male sex hormones
> Sulphonamides – anti-bacterial
> Chlorpromazine (e.g. Largactil) tranquillizers
> Phenytoin (Epanutin) – used to control epilepsy
> Carbamazepine (Tegretol) – used to treat epilepsy and trigeminal neuralgia
> Levodopa (Sinemet) – Parkinson's disease

5) Deficiency or Excess of Iodine

In 1960 estimates showed that 200 million people worldwide suffered iodine-deficient hypothyroidism.

Iodine is a trace mineral found in the soil and in our food. The richest food sources are in seafood and seaweed. Most of the body's iodine is in the thyroid. A deficiency in iodine can result in a compensatory swelling of the thyroid known as a goitre.

Iodine is an essential component of the hormones T_4 and T_3 and the numbers relate to the number of iodine atoms in each hormone.

Paradoxically, an excess of iodine, whether dietary (caused by eating too much seafood), or overzealous supplementation, can inactivate production of the thyroid hormones leading to enlargement or goitre. A goitre can therefore result from both an under and an overactive thyroid condition.

The recommended dietary allowance (RDA) is 100mcg for women and 120mcg for men. However, a daily intake of up to 1000 mcg would not harm a healthy thyroid.

The Japanese with their diet of seafood, dulse kelp and sea lettuce tolerate daily intakes of iodine of around 400,000–500,000 mcg. Not surprisingly, the inland and mountainous regions of the world, well away from the seas and oceans constitute the main iodine deficient areas.

In iodine deficient areas, animals also suffer thyroid deficiencies:

> Sheep produce less wool.
> Cattle become sterile and have a lower milk yield.
> Hens' eggs lack calcium and break easily.
> Horses become lethargic and work-shy.

6) Secondary Causes

Pituitary or Hypothalamic Problems

The pituitary gland controls the thyroid, and the hypothalamus in the brain controls the pituitary. Functional deficiencies or imbalances in the two areas can reduce thyroid efficiency.

7) Cancer

Cancer of the throat and other areas of the neck adjacent to the thyroid, can adversely influence the circulation and hence the nutrition to the gland. Many other types of cancer will depress metabolic efficiency, and this can reduce the thyroid hormone output. The activity of the thyroid can reflect the metabolism in many ways. When it is possible to cure any chronic illness the thyroid usually normalizes.

8) Poor Conversion of T₄ to T₃

One of the chief areas of controversy surrounding the diagnosis and treatment of hypothyroidism is the conversion of T_4 (thyroxine) to T_3 (triiodothyronine). As I mentioned on page 10 T_3 is more active than T_4 and is in fact four times more potent; although our blood contains 50 times more T_4 than T_3. The metabolism of the conversion of T_4 to T_3 takes place chiefly in the liver, but all phases of the production and release of the two thyroid hormones are under the control of the thyroid stimulating hormone (TSH) released by the pituitary gland. It is possible that in many cases of hypothyroidism, the conversion of the T_4 to T_3 is impaired as a result of enzyme failure, free radical damage or liver toxicity.

If this poor conversion is the cause of the depressed thyroid, simply prescribing extra T_4 may not be the answer. Many doctors in the USA are now using a combined T_4/T_3 protocol. In the UK T_4 alone is prescribed on the basis that patients' metabolism should convert T_4 to T_3 as needed. However 20 per cent of T_3 is produced directly from the thyroid, so a T_3 deficit can easily develop with hypothyroidism even when plenty of T_4 is available.

Dr Arem who is chief of Endocrinology at Ben Taub General Hospital in America has observed that when he changed his patients' prescriptions from whole desiccated thyroid to thyroxine, patients complained of symptoms returning. 'This was in spite of having reached normal blood levels of thyroid hormones and TSH'. This concept of poor T^4 to T^3 conversion offers a plausable rationale for prescribing whole animal thyroid for mild hypothyroidism.

Other Causes of Subclinical Hypothyroidism

If we recognize that there are degrees of thyroid malfunction, it follows that there are likely to be degrees of severity when considering the causes.

As with many functional health disorders, the symptoms can be the end result of a large number of different causes. Although for the physician it is always easier to diagnose and treat when there is only a single cause to consider, with mild hypothyroidism, many layers of causes may exist. These combine to produce the characteristic symptoms that serve to provide the evidence for diagnosis.

Subclinical or mild hypothyroidism can cause many symptoms, but conversely many factors can cause the thyroid to become less efficient. Perhaps the great number and variety of causes listed below serves to explain the increasing prevalence of this problem.

Let us now look at some of the 'unofficial' causes of hypothyroidism.

Almost any illness, trauma or circumstance that depresses the metabolism has the potential to also depress the thyroid. This may be a transient reaction lasting for two to three weeks, or a lifelong response with irreversible thyroid collapse.

In common with many health problems, there are very often several factors involved in causing hypothyroidism.

The eight groups of causes already discussed are in general easy to recognize and usually involve major health changes. The many less obvious factors that I shall now outline, that contribute to mild hypothyroidism are not so easily identified, for several reasons. The great diversity of the causes probably contributes to the frequent mis-diagnosis of this common health problem.

Other reasons for a missed diagnosis can include:

* The causes may appear too trivial to influence the thyroid gland.
* With many of the causes there is no obvious connection with the thyroid.
* Many causes are so commonplace that their potential to disturb the thyroid is not appreciated or recognized.
* It is very easy to attribute symptoms to other health problems, and the thyroid involvement can be missed.

Other Causes

1   Pregnancy – (post-partum thyrotoxicosis)
2   Candidiasis
3   Spinal injury (RTA – whiplash injury)
4   Surgery (adjacent neck surgery)
5   The results of infection – e.g. post-viral fatigue (PVF), glandular fever (mononucleosis) and ME (myalgic-encephalomyelitis)
6   Stress
7   Menopause
8   Nutritional deficiencies
     Protein deficiency (e.g. glutathione and tyrosine)
     B vitamins deficiency
     Vitamin A, vitamin C and vitamin E deficiencies
     Deficiency of the minerals copper, zinc, iron, manganese and selenium.
9   Goitregens in food
10 Mercury amalgam in dental fillings
11 Adrenal hypofunction
12 Anorexia nervosa and bulimia
13 Leaky gut and malabsorption
14 The liver
15 Heredity
16 Tobacco

17   Fluoridation of water
18   Essential fatty acid deficiency

These causes of mild hypothyroidism fall naturally into four main groups.

A) Endocrine Causes

Disturbances to the endocrine axis. The other glands on the axis can influence the thyroid.

B) Local Causes

Disturbance to the local neck structures including the vertebrae, the nerves or the blood flow, can all adversely influence and suppress the thyroid function.

C) General Causes

Almost anything that disturbs the metabolic tempo of the body has the potential to depress the thyroid.

D) Non Specific Causes

This is a wide list including toxic substances and deficiencies.

1) Pregnancy and the Thyroid

During pregnancy, the thyroid gland can increase in volume by up to 25 or 30 per cent in order to enable the woman's metabolism to deal with the changes that occur as the baby grows. This enlargement is partly caused by hormone changes, but other factors include the loss of iodine in the urine that occurs with pregnancy, and the baby taking the mother's iodine. This highlights the need for an adequate intake of iodine by the mother by taking supplements, eating regular seafood or the use of iodized salt.

Post-partum thyroiditis (PPT)

This is an auto-immune problem. The pregnant mother's immune system is normally depressed to reduce the risk of rejection of the foetus. This can lead to the immune system becoming confused, and one subsequent result of this is inflammation of the thyroid. Up to 10 per cent of women have the potential to develop PPT, which can worsen after the baby is born. Significantly, although this condition usually improves spontaneously without treatment, many women (up to 40 per cent) tend to develop long-term hypothyroidism within 12 months following the birth. It is not uncommon for PPT to occur up to three to four years after the birth. All this means that when pregnancy disturbs and depresses the thyroid, the gland can be weakened for several years. An important consideration with diagnosis.

Early and accurate diagnosis of thyroid imbalance during pregnancy is of particular importance for a variety of reasons.

1) A reduced level of thyroid in the early stages of pregnancy can influence development of the baby's brain leading to cretinism.

2) Miscarriages in early pregnancy are often a result of hypothyroidism.

As hypothyroidism can lead to infertility, severe thyroid deficiencies in pregnancy are rare. The diagnosis of chronic infertility should always include a full blood thyroid screen.

2) Candidiasis (thrush)

Candida albicans is a yeast that is present in the gastrointestinal tract of all of us. When the yeast colony is controlled, no symptoms arise. If, however, there occurs a yeast overgrowth then a wide range of symptoms can develop. This condition is termed 'the yeast syndrome' or chronic candidiasis. The body systems particularly vulnerable to candidiasis include the genito-urinary, gastrointestinal, immune and endocrine systems. With severe candidiasis (e.g. as in AIDS patients), the central nervous system can also be diseased. Food intolerances and food allergies have also been linked to this condition as the candida can cause 'leaky gut syndrome' which is believed to be a major cause of food intolerances.

The Causes

Chronic candidiasis is caused by a variety of factors, these include:

1   Antibiotic use. The beneficial gut bacteria which normally help to control candida are destroyed by antibiotics. (This is termed dysbiosis.)
2   Steroid drugs
3   Drugs prescribed for stomach ulcers and inflammation (gastritis)

4   Oral contraceptives
5   High sugar diets
6   Diabetes
7   Leaky gut (Faulty absorption through the gut wall.)
8   Digestive enzyme deficiency
9   Faulty liver function
10 A constitutional or acquired immune deficiency
11 Environmental influences including stress, pollution, chemicals and general poor nutrition.
12 Endocrine system exhaustion

It is the last cause in the list that is relevant to this book. It has been known for many years that our immune system and our stress-handling system are both weakened when the thyroid is underactive.

The chronic candidiasis–endocrine link was highlighted by Dr Phyliss Saiffer MD during a conference held in 1985. She defined the candida-induced exhaustion of the endocrine glands as Autoimmune disease, Polyendocrinopathy Immune-dysregulation Candidiasis and Hypersensitivity – APICH for short.

She outlined nine key conditions that can result from candidiasis-induced immune suppression. These being:

1   Hypothyroidism
2   Autoimmune thyroidosis (Hashimoto's and Graves disease)
3   Hypoadrenalism (adrenal exhaustion)
4   Diabetes
5   Hypoparathyroidism – causing calcium depletion and tetany. The parathyroids consist of a group of lobed glands adjacent to the thyroid. They secrete a hormone which helps to maintain the level of blood calcium concentration.
6   Pernicious anaemia. Reduced vitamin B_{12} absorption, resulting from a lowered secretion of the 'intrinsic factor' which is produced in the stomach to facilitate absorption of vitamin B_{12}.

7   Hepatitis – inflammation of the liver
8   Alopecia – loss of hair
9   Vitiligo – whitening of skin areas

Many other conditions have been attributed to the effects of candidiasis on our hormones. These include allergies, muscle weakness, PMS, IBS (irritable bowel syndrome), SLE (system lupus erythematosis), rheumatoid arthritis and autism.

JUDITH'S STORY

Judith had worked as a hairdresser for 32 years, eventually owning and managing her own successful salon. She had suffered with dry eczema on her hands and arms most of her life, but the symptoms had been minimized with the occasional application of steroid cream and the avoidance of cows' milk products.

THE HISTORY

Her skin problem had developed during puberty and Judith was advised to consult an allergist. Tests had shown an intolerance to cows' milk and any food or drink that contained cows' milk. Fortunately, Judith was quite happy to rely on goat and sheep's milk products. So apart from a slight worsening during the winter, and temporary flare-ups following stress, the eczema appeared to be well under control.

All this had changed two years ago, when following a severe bout of cystitis, for which several courses of antibiotics were prescribed, Judith developed candida (thrush). This was followed by intestinal symptoms including diarrhoea, bloating and discomfort. Her doctor defined these symptoms as IBS and prescribed antacids and drugs for bowel frequency.

THE RAPID WORSENING

Shortly after this Judith experienced a worsening of the eczema. The skin on the hands became very dry, with splitting, and subsequently bleeding occurred. The nails also cracked and split. She had always been very proud of her strong shapely nails and her skin was usually clear enough for her condition to pass unnoticed when working. Her clients now commented on the state of her hands and she was very distressed by the appearance of her skin, and the discomfort to her hands when working.

THE WORK AND STRESS

For the first time in her career, the chemicals that Judith had used every day in her work without any adverse side effects, were now aggravating her hands and causing inflammation and itching. She was obliged to wear protective gloves to reduce her embarrassment and to prevent a worsening of the eczema.

She reduced her work load and was obliged to hire extra staff. This placed a strain on her finances, and in little over a year her business – which had always been profitable – became a financial liability and she faced bankruptcy.

THE CONSULTATION

Judith consulted me around 18 months after the cystitis and IBS problems, by which time she had become very anxious and depressed. Furthermore, although previously a vital, alert and happy woman, she had slipped into a state of chronic fatigue. Her memory and concentration had become blurred and unreliable, and this additional source of stress was probably aggravating her eczema.

Judith had entered a vicious circle of cause and effect so characteristic of patients with a low grade or mild hypothyroidism. A typical pattern is shown below.

THE VICIOUS CIRCLE

Mild hypothyroidism

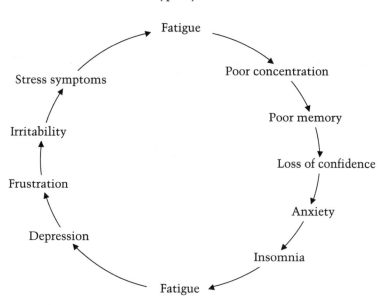

Fatigue
Poor concentration
Poor memory
Loss of confidence
Anxiety
Insomnia
Fatigue
Depression
Frustration
Irritability
Stress symptoms

Alongside the fatigue and skin breakdown, Judith was experiencing several other symptoms. These included a continuous body coldness. Paradoxically she also suffered hot flushes, three to four times every night. Another great concern to her was a recent tendency to hair loss. As a hairdresser she was aware of the normal rate of hair loss, and she knew that her loss of hair was becoming excessive.

THE TESTING

I requested a set of blood tests. These included a biochemistry screen, a haematology screen, a serum mineral profile and a thyroid profile. The results showed that Judith was deficient in chromium, zinc and magnesium. The biochemistry showed raised levels of cholesterol and triglycerides. The haematology was normal but the thyroid hormones were at the lower end of the normal range. Upon booking her consultation, Judith had been requested to check her early morning temperatures for one week. These showed an average temperature of 97.2°F (36.2°C).

THE TREATMENT

The case histories in this book are essentially typical cases of mild hypothyroidism. However, the thyroid influences many organs and systems in the body, so inevitably the effects of an underactive thyroid feature in many health problems.

Although Judith presented fairly typical symptoms of a mildly underactive thyroid she had related problems that needed treatment. These included:

1   Mineral deficiencies.
    Zinc is essential for skin health and repair. Magnesium is a key component in energy production.
    Many patients with chronic fatigue syndrome show low magnesium when tested. Chromium is also known as the 'glucose tolerance factor' and plays a vital role in the blood sugar balance.
    Judith had low levels of all these minerals.

2   Hormonal imbalance.
    The thyroid gland is closely involved in the balance of other glands that form the endocrine axis. These include the adrenal and the ovarian glands. Judith's hot flushes suggested a perimenopausal state induced by a depressed oestrogen level. Her chronic worsening stress was causing adrenal exhaustion, poor stress handling and anxiety.

3   Poor skin health.
    Skin health and repair is dependent upon many nutrients. It would be quite wrong to attribute all Judith's symptoms to a

poor thyroid efficiency. When a condition becomes chronic (i.e. long-term) other associated problems need to be treated.

4   Chronic antibiotic induced candidiasis.
     As outlined above, the role of candidiasis in contributing to mild hypothyroidism is well recognized.
     Judith was prescribed glandular extract for adrenal, ovarian and thyroid support. A full anti-candida programme was provided, including a yeast and sugar free diet, multi-minerals and vitamins including zinc, chromium, magnesium and vitamin A and B complex and fish oils to improve the skin health. A low animal fat, sugar-free diet was also recommended.

THE PROGRESS

Within six weeks Judith began to regain her previous energy levels and in three months her skin was repaired and was looking and feeling much healthier.

The ovarian/adrenal support had reduced the hot flushes to a very occasional episode at night.

After six months of treatment, Judith had returned to full-time work. Her latest blood test showed that her thyroid hormones were near the middle of the normal range and her morning temperatures were averaging 97.8°F (36.6°C).

It is of value to note that many of the symptoms associated with APICH are also common to hypothyroidism. In particular fatigue, postnatal depression, food and chemical sensitivities, muscle pain, anxiety and depression, menstrual irregularities and infertility.

3) Spinal Injuries

As an osteopath, I am frequently requested to treat spinal symptoms that have developed as a result of road traffic accidents, surgery and dental treatment, skiing, horse riding accidents and contact sport injuries (e.g. rugby). These symptoms are usually located in the neck region. Whiplash injuries as a result of motor accidents can inflict considerable strain, muscle damage and loss of the normal neck curve. This is termed a 'reversed curve' which often requires the use of a remedial pillow and long-term treatment. Unfortunately, when there is an absence of fracture or obvious damage, many accident victims are sent home with a prescription for pain killing drugs. There is evidence however that whip-lash and similar injuries can disturb the nerves and blood vessels that supply the thyroid, causing the gland to become gradually less efficient.

SALLY'S STORY

THE ACCIDENT

Following the motor accident that killed her husband, Sally was unconscious with head injuries for four weeks. In addition to the concussion she suffered whip-lash symptoms, lacerations and severe bruising to the head and shoulders. Fortunately there were no fractures, so Sally was able to return home two months later. Her remaining symptoms being a recurring frontal headache, neck and shoulder stiffness and numbness in the right arm and leg.

THE SYMPTOMS

Before the accident Sally was an energetic, slim 56 year old housewife. When she consulted me a little over a year after leaving hospital, she had changed in many ways.

Her weight had increased by 25lb and she was suffering with exhaustion. With the loving support of her three children she had retained her optimism, and although her husband's death had left a great gap in her life, she was not depressed. However, she did have difficulty keeping warm, particularly at night. This was never a problem prior to the accident. Her fatigue deterred her from exercising and her increased weight was causing her to be breathless. She also noticed that coffee, alcohol and sugar caused her heart to race. Her blood pressure was too high for her age.

Sally was beginning to lose her self-confidence and was concerned that she looked 'fat and old'.

THE DIAGNOSIS

She had discussed her symptoms with the hospital consultants and her own doctor. She was told that the fatigue was caused by the shock and trauma of the accident, coupled with the excess weight. Reassurance was given that with time and careful dieting, she would regain her health and energy. Her weight increase was put down to comfort eating resulting from bereavement. This view was a little unfair as Sally had discussed her diet with the hospital nutritionist, and she usually consumed no more than 1500 calories each day.

The other symptoms including the raised blood pressure and reactions to coffee, sugar and alcohol were attributed to the weight increase.

There is an increasingly common tendency in medical diagnosis to attribute symptoms to such causes as weight, stress, age or even one's gender. Doctors frequently settle for this explanation when tests are inconclusive or they feel unable to make a precise diagnosis. This leads them to either blame the patient ... 'you must lose weight before you can feel well', or to blame circumstances 'you must expect these problems now that you are 50' or 'what do you expect, you are a woman?'.

CAUSES AND SYMPTOMS

In my experience, pain, excess weight, fatigue, depression and many other symptoms are by definition symptoms and not usually the causes of ill health. With this in mind the symptoms can only be resolved when the true causes are identified and effectively treated.

For Sally, the causes of her symptoms had yet to be identified. Routine hospital blood tests for anaemia, diabetes and heart and kidney function had all shown normal results. Hence the diagnosis of 'post-traumatic stress' and 'comfort eating'. Sally knew that victims of road traffic accidents do not usually suffer exhaustion and obesity. She came to see me convinced that her metabolism had somehow changed as a result of the accident.

THE CONSULTATION

Her weight at her consultation was 156lb, and with a height of 5ft and medium sized hands and feet, I considered that she was 30lb overweight. I requested a morning temperature test and a thyroid profile blood test.

Sally's average temperature over four days was 96.6°F (35.8°C) and her blood showed a very low level of thyroid activity.

I considered it likely that her weight and fatigue resulted from her underactive thyroid, with the raised blood pressure and palpitations being secondary symptoms.

The thyroid is involved in the control of other glands, including the adrenal glands, and hypothyroidism, particularly when coupled with stress, can lead to adrenal exhaustion. One of the many roles of the adrenal glands is to release adrenalin to increase blood sugar levels. The body's ability to fine-tune any sudden falls in the blood sugar can be compromised, and the insulin–adrenalin balance is disturbed. When this occurs, caffeine, alcohol and sugar can cause inappropriate and disturbing fluctuations in the blood sugar levels.

THE TREATMENT

Sally was prescribed a maximum dosage of thyroid glandular extract and her blood was retested after three months. The thyroid and pituitary hormones were well into the normal range although towards the lower end, but another test after six months showed satisfactory levels of all the hormones.

Over the following six months Sally's weight fell to 140lb and her vitality and wellbeing were much improved. Her blood pressure remained slightly raised but her palpitations cleared.

TRAUMA AND THE THYROID

When the blood flow to the thyroid gland is disturbed the thyroid can malfunction. Adjacent injury or surgery can be a cause. It seems very likely that Sally's whip-lash injury and the throat and neck bruising depressed her thyroid function, and the thyroid glandular treatment normalized the imbalance.

4) Surgery

Mild post-surgical hypothyroidism is a well recognized problem. The metabolic rate can be depressed for three to four months following a general anaesthetic. In addition, the anaethetist requires the patient's head to be flexed backwards. This can cause the neck structure to be stressed. It is not unusual for patients to complain of neck symptoms following surgery.

When I am consulted by a patient with suspected mild hypothyroidism, I always inquire about past traumas, spinal symptoms and surgery. There is often a gap of several years between cause and symptoms, so it is essential that a patient's whole life be reviewed.

I have seen mention of an unproven hypothesis that the thyroid may be disturbed with birth trauma e.g. forceps delivery. This has yet to be confirmed.

Dental Treatment

Heavy one-sided dental extractions and other dental treatments have been known to strain the cervical vertebrae. This has lead to a re-designing of dental equipment and techniques in recent years to minimize the risk of such occurrences.

Adjacent surgery to the thyroid e.g. tonsillectomy is also suspected as a possible cause of mild hypothyroidism. It is assumed that the thyroid function is disturbed following surgery. Fortunately this type of problem is usually transient and short-term, and such operations are no longer fashionable following the discovery of antibiotics.

5) Infections, Post-Viral Fatigue (PVF) and ME

It is well recognized that mild hypothyroidism can depress the immune system. Many practitioners and researchers consider that the majority of the symptoms of PVF and ME are caused by an underactive thyroid.

The British Thyroid Foundation are currently encouraging British doctors to prescribe very low dose thyroxine

> for patients with chronic fatigue. Dr Gordon Skinner
> claims up to 65 per cent improvement over a three
> month period. He has appealed to colleagues in a letter
> to the *British Medical Journal* to embrace the concept of
> mild hypothyroidism[1].

Patients often tell me that they have been fatigued since a bout of 'flu, a chest infection, cystitis, or other types of infections. These past infections often occur up to three years previously. They have usually been given the vague diagnosis of post-viral fatigue with little or no treatment offered. The term myalgic encphalomyelitis (ME) has been largely superseded by the term chronic fatigue syndrome. CFS is perhaps even more vague than post-viral fatigue (PVF), as it only describes the symptoms. However, all three terms describe a similar group of symptoms. I find that the majority of such patients have low basal temperatures and abnormally low levels of thyroid hormones. Furthermore they usually show a good response to thyroid treatment. I am convinced that when fatigue and other symptoms follow an infection, the first and most rewarding step should be to assess the thyroid.

Following infections the whole metabolism can be left depressed and underactive. This specifically applies to the thyroid, and appropriate treatment can often reverse what has happened.

> As stated elsewhere in this book, routine blood tests are
> usually not sensitive enough to identify mild levels of
> hypothyroidism. However, patients with symptoms of
> PVF, ME or CFS invariably show blood tests results at
> the lower end of the normal ranges. Significantly, following
> treatment, the thyroid results improve as their
> symptoms improve.

6) Stress

Many health writers and practitioners succumb to the temptation to blame health problems on stress. We hear that stress can cause cancer, arthritis, asthma, diabetes, allergies, IBS depression, fatigue etc. It is a very long list of complaints.

If we accept that stress plays a major role in our health, what exactly links the mind and body and what can we do about reducing the harmful effects of stress? Why does news of a disaster in the media cause one person to burst into tears and become depressed, while another person seems unaffected and indifferent? The stress potential itself does not vary, so the key would appear to be our own ability to deal with the stress. This surely depends on our interpretation of, and our response to the stress. Some see our ability to deal with a crisis as a combination of strength of personality, courage and experience. In fact, it is more likely that our ability to deal with any type of stress depends on our stamina, our experience and our adrenal efficiency.

Unfortunately there is still a tendency in 20th century medicine to separate the mind from the body. Many depressed, anxious patients are referred to psychologists or psychiatrists, when they would probably derive greater benefit from consulting a naturopath or a nutritionist. The mind and body work together. Every thought involves a chemical activity in our brain. Subtle changes in brain chemistry can alter our personality.

This concept is well demonstrated in the aggressive alcoholic, the personality changes caused by LSD and other drugs, and the well recognized influence of PMS on many women's behaviour. Post-natal depression and many cases of schizophrenia have also been linked to nutritional deficiencies and blood sugar swings. The diabetic who 'hypos' when he or she overdoses on insulin becomes aggressive and unsociable. This is not a personality defect, but a transient reversible and fairly minor fall in the blood sugar level.

The adrenal system is our stress-handling control. Chronic or

long-term stress of any kind has the potential to exhaust the adrenals. When this occurs the whole endocrine axis can be depressed,
including the thyroid. It is generally accepted that people under
stress are more prone to suffer infections. The immune system is
weakened by stress through the influence of stress on the thyroid
gland, and the adrenal glands.

7) Menopause and Perimenopause

Many women develop a mildly underactive thyroid prior to
menopause. (This time is known as the perimenopausal period and
can occur several years before periods cease.)

When this occurs there is a tendency to begin early menopausal
symptoms. These can include missed periods and hot flushes. It is
thought that the hormonal changes that precede the menopause contribute to the thyroid deficiency. Certainly the symptoms of mild
hypothyroidism are very similar. These include fatigue, depression,
weight increase and headaches. Unfortunately, many doctors tend to
assume that the symptoms are entirely menopausal, and as a result,
the thyroid involvement can be missed.

Just as any existing thyroid deficiency can worsen with the
menopause, menopause can depress the thyroid so a vicious circle
is established. This can only be effectively resolved when the thyroid is also treated, alongside any support needed for the female
hormones.

8) Nutritional Deficiencies

We do not eat hormones. Adrenalin, thyroxine, insulin and oestrogen are not found in our food, they have to be manufactured. Our
wonderfully complex body chemistry synthesizes many nutrients
to make the hormones. Thyroxine is composed of the amino acid

(protein constituent) tyrosine and the mineral iodine. Whilst tyrosine is itself converted from the amino acid phenylalamine. It is therefore logical to assume that the production of thyroxine will be compromised in proportion to any deficiency of tyrosine and/or iodine.

As tyrosine is a protein constituent, anything that adversely affects protein metabolism has the potential to reduce tyrosine levels. This includes chronic disease (e.g. cancer, hepatitis, Kwashiorkor), low protein diets (e.g. anorexia, veganism) or the results of poverty. Unfortunately, protein foods tend to be costly to produce and purchase. Very low income groups therefore chiefly rely on carbohydrates, including rice, cereals, potatoes etc. Any diet that serves to minimize the intake of the essential vitamins, minerals and proteins that are required for normal thyroid function, can encourage or worsen mild hypothyroidism. In this context diets that are low in certain nutrients have been linked to hypothyroidism. These nutrients include vitamins, minerals and proteins.

Vitamins

VITAMIN A
Although one's diet may be rich in the carotenes (the orange coloured substances the body normally converts to vitamin A), a vitamin A deficiency can still occur as an underactive thyroid can suppress the conversion rate. Typical symptoms of vitamin A deficiency include poor night vision, yellow skin (caused by the unconverted beta carotene) and poor protein use. Therefore a deficiency of vitamin A can reduce protein availability and use in the body. This is shown strikingly in Kwashiorkor, a common condition found mainly in South America, Africa and India, that is caused by a severe protein deficiency.

The English author Isobel W. Jennings wrote in 1970 that deficiency of vitamin A in animal feed affected their ability to produce TSH (thyroid stimulating hormone)[2]. This occurs in sheep and cattle as a result of pituitary degeneration.

Danish research has shown a fall in pigs' thyroid production of up to 50 per cent when vitamin A was removed from their diet. This occurring after only two weeks.

Conversely, experiments involving the removal of rabbits' thyroids caused bulging eyes (exophthalmos), usually associated with hyperthyroidism. Significantly beta carotene did not improve the condition, but Vitamin A administration resolved all the symptoms. Vitamin A is also required for the effective conversion of the hormone T_4 to T_3.

THE B VITAMINS

The exact role of many nutrients in thyroid function is so subtle and complex that it is only by the close study of deficiency symptoms, usually artificially produced in laboratory animals, or seen in severe human deficiency diseases, that the cause and effect link can be predictably demonstrated.

VITAMIN B1 (THIAMINE)

Although not directly linked to hypothyroidism, a vitamin B_1 deficiency can cause very similar symptoms to a depressed thyroid. Supplementing hypothyroid patients with B_1 has improved their memory, mood and concentration.

VITAMIN B2 (RIBOFLAVIN)

Essential for conversion of the amino acid phenylalanine to tyrosine. A deficiency of B_2 can also block the production and release of the pituitary hormone TSH.

VITAMIN B12

An essential vitamin for conversion of phenylalanine to tyrosine. Rats deprived of their thyroids cannot absorb B_{12}. Blood B_{12} deficiency in humans improves with thyroid treatment.

FOLIC ACID

Another essential vitamin in thyroid metabolism. Folic acid is a co-factor alongside vitamin C and copper in tyrosine metabolism (see proteins below).

VITAMIN C

Guinea pigs, like humans, cannot synthesize vitamin C from food, so are required to consume it. Consequently when deficient in vitamin C they can develop capillary damage (small blood vessel damage), with subsequent bleeding into the thyroid tissue. Vitamin C with copper and folic acid is involved in the metabolism of tyrosine (see proteins below).

VITAMIN E

An essential vitamin to allow conversion of phenylalanine to tyrosine. Rabbits with induced vitamin E deficiency, also show reduced TSH synthesis.

Minerals

SELENIUM

Selenium plays an essential role in the conversion of T_4 to T_3. It also protects against free radical damage. Tissue levels of selenium reduce with age and this mineral is usually deficient in soils that have been intensively worked.

MANGANESE

Manganese assists the transport of T_4 and is involved in thyroxine production.

COPPER

Copper is essential for the conversion of T_4 to T_3 at cellular level. In hypothyroidism, copper absorption by the gastrointestinal tract can be reduced. It also plays a role in tyrosine metabolism (see proteins below).

ZINC

Zinc is needed for the efficient conversion of T_4 to T_3. Animals deficient in zinc can suffer thyroid damage. Tissue zinc levels reduce with age and can be deficient in Down's syndrome. When zinc is prescribed the thyroid hormone levels usually improve.

IRON

Iron is essential for the conversion of phenylalanine to tyrosine. However, overzealous supplementation of iron can cause an excess of tyrosine which can bind thyroid hormones and reduces absorption.

ANTIOXIDANTS

The chief role of natural antioxidants is to neutralize and make harmless the free radicals. Free radicals are toxic substances, they are formed as a by-product of oxygen consumption. They can damage cells and seriously disturb the body's immune efficiency.

> Synthetic antioxidants are added to many foods, paints, oils, rubbers etc., to prevent or delay the deterioration of the substance by the action of the oxygen in the air.

The chief natural antioxidants are vitamins A, C, E and selenium. They are all discussed above and all generally support the health of the thyroid.

Proteins

You will recall that several amino acids (the building blocks of proteins) are involved in thyroid metabolism. These include:

CARNITINE

The value of carnitine in treating hypothyroidism has yet to be proven. However, studies have shown that carnitine metabolism is depressed in hypothyroidism and normalized when the thyroid is treated.

Patients with low adrenal, thyroid and pituitary activity have been found to be deficient in serum (blood) carnitine.

GLUTATHIONE

This substance which is made up of three amino acids: cysteine, glutamine and glycine, is also involved in thyroid function. It works as an antioxidant and alongside the vitamins A, C and E, the mineral selenium and the other amino acids methionine and cysteine, helps control free radical activity.

TYROSINE

This important amino acid is the precursor of T_3 and T_4. When the iodine levels are normal, supplementary tyrosine can improve thyroid activity. A mild serum tyrosine deficiency has been observed with hypothyroid patients. Tyrosine is also successfully prescribed in the treatment of depression.

PHENYLALANINE

While tyrosine is the precursor of the thyroid hormones, it is itself derived from phenylalanine. Deficiency of the enzyme which is required by the metabolism to convert phenylalanine to tyrosine, (phenylalanine hydroxylase), results in PKU (phenylketonuria). The subsequent deficiency of tyrosine and excess of phenylalanine reduces thyroid activity.

Fatigue, obesity and poor immunity are some of the symptoms that result.

When the two forms of phenylalanine are combined (d and l) the resulting mixture is known as DLPA. One of the major uses of DLPA is for pain relief; it prolongs the life of the brain endorphins that have an analgesic role.

9) Goitregens

Iodine deficiency is now relatively unknown in Western industrial nations. This is largely as a result of adding iodine to animal feed and table salt. Unfortunately, in areas where the pre-existing iodine consumption was adequate, the extra 'added' iodine has lead to an increase in hyperthyroidism.

In spite of the value of iodine supplementation being identified in the 1930s the incidence of thyroid goitres has **not** reduced. The current figures are five to six per cent of the population in certain parts of the US.

Many researchers believe that the figures are the result of eating foods that reduce iodine uptake by the thyroid. These are known as Goitregens. So named because eating them can lead to goitre formation and thyroid underactivity. Their influence is caused by cyanide derivatives contained in the plants, and a substance named goitrin.

Before becoming too concerned you can be reassured that when moderation and variety is practised in one's diet, goitregens can be safely eaten. Economically enforced lack of variety in one's diet, and the use of mono-diets and 'special diets' by enthusiasts can lead to risk.

A further reassurance is the fact that goitregens are usually inactivated with cooking. As can be noted from the list that follows, these foods are rarely eaten uncooked (perhaps with the exception of nuts).

Goitregens

Vegetables

Mainly cruciferous plants of the brassica (mustard) family and including: Cabbage, cauliflower, kohlrabi, sprouts, kale, swede, turnip, mustard and rape.

Others include cassava, and soya.

Cereals

Maize or sweet corn and millet (also including millet flour or sorghum).

Nuts

Peanuts, pine nuts, almonds and walnuts.

Seeds

Mustard and rape seeds.

The goitregens need only to be considered as a risk factor when these foods form a major part of one's diet.

The influence of goitregens (in the brassica family), was shown clearly in Tasmania in 1949. After an increase in goitres in school children, iodine tablets were supplied. The goitres did not improve, in fact the numbers increased. In the same year a free school milk programme had started, and farmers were obliged to feed their cattle on kale to meet the extra demand. Kale is a member of the brassica family, and the goitregenic compound contained in the kale passed into the children's milk and blocked use of the iodine in the tablets.[3]

10) Mercury Amalgam

There is evidence available to show that mercury, mainly introduced into our systems from dental amalgam, has an adverse effect on thyroid function. Various researchers have demonstrated over the last 40 years that exposure to mercury can depress animal thyroids, often irreversibly. Mercury amalgam has been used in dentistry for 150 years. Many specialist dentists are currently removing mercury amalgam from thousands of patients for a variety of reasons. It is likely that we will hear more information in the future on the mercury–thyroid link.

> The removal of amalgam fillings is a controversial subject within the dental profession. The amalgam consists of several metals, including silver, copper, mercury and tin. Although research results are inconclusive, sensitive individuals claim improvement in their health with amalgam removal. A variety of conditions have been linked to mercury in fillings including ME, IBS, diabetes, rheumatoid arthritis, lupus (SLE) and hypothyroidism. Naturopaths and nutritionists point to the value of taking the antioxident nutrients which serve to reduce mercury in the body. These include the minerals selenium, zinc and copper, and the vitamins A, C and E. Significantly, autopsies carried out on dentists have shown high concentrations of mercury in their pituitary glands. The pituitary is the control gland for the thyroid.

11) Underactive Adrenal Glands (Hypo-adrenalism)

Stress can lead to adrenal exhaustion. This can influence thyroid efficiency by various pathways. These include:

* The amino acid tyrosine is one of the precursors for the thyroid hormones and the adrenal hormones. When the adrenal glands are over functioning as a response to chronic stress, the tyrosine requirements are stepped up at the expense of thyroid function.
* Many of the vitamins, minerals, trace elements and proteins required for optimum thyroid function are also depleted with adrenal stress. These include the B complex vitamins, zinc, selenium and especially vitamin C.
* The high level of adrenal hormones found in the blood as a direct response to stress, can reduce the efficient conversion of T_4 to T_3. Adrenal exhaustion or hypoadrenalism as a result of chronic stress, is seen as an increasingly common cause of mild hypothyroidism.

12) Anorexia Nervosa and Bulimia

Anorexia involves virtual self-starvation. This problem, which is usually found amongst teenage girls has psycho-physiological components of self-image and weight fear. However, research has shown that taste perception plays a leading role, as anorexic patients find it very difficult to taste bitter or sour flavours. This can be caused by a zinc deficiency. Zinc supplementation has been found to improve the appetite of anorexic patients, which plays a vital role in their rehabilitation.

Bulimia

This condition involves 'bingeing'. The word bulimia meaning literally 'ox hunger'. To avoid obesity many bulimic patients deliberately vomit shortly after eating. Lack of periods (amenorrhoea) is often present with bulimia. As with anorexia, a nutritional programme including zinc supplementation has been shown to be helpful.

Both these disorders present a challenge to the body's normal rate of metabolism. The weight loss with anorexia, and the cessation of periods and frequent vomiting in bulimia suggest nutrient deficiencies are present, not least zinc which I have already discussed. Zinc deficiency can influence thyroid efficiency. The hormone leptrin may be the link between anorexia, bulimia and mild hypothyroidism. In his book *The Thyroid Solution* Dr Ridha Arem states 'Leptrin promotes a reduced caloric intake and an increase in the metabolic rate. When you do not eat for a long period of time, leptrin levels decrease and lead to changes in the endocrine system that result in reduced metabolism – when the potent thyroid hormone T_3 is not delivered in sufficient amounts, leptrin becomes inefficient in enhancing metabolism'[3].

This may well lead to a vicious circle of depressed metabolic rate, low thyroid output and further metabolic depression.

As I have already described the thyroid sets the pace for our metabolism but conversely, changes to our metabolism can alter the thyroid. Anorexia and bulimia are two health problems that can stress a young person's metabolic efficiency. The weight loss of anorexia and the vomiting and bingeing of bulimia, when experienced by a body still growing and developing, is liable to destabilize thyroid efficiency and depress output of the vital thyroid hormones.

13) Leaky Gut and Malabsorption

I regularly request an intestinal permeability test. This simple, valuable test that patients carry out in their own home involves taking a very small amount of polyethylene glycol 400 (or PEG), as a flavourless drink.

This substance consists of a mixture of 11 different sized moleculars. These pass through the gut wall, into the circulation and eventually into the bladder. A six hour total urine measurement following ingestion of the PEG is made, and the amount of each of the 11 molecules passed is measured in the laboratory. When compared with the normal ranges, an absorption profile is constructed and a graph is produced. If too much of the polyethylene is passed, a leaky gut is suspected. If too little, there may be malabsorption as a result of mucus or toxins in the gut.

> A leaky gut can cause local symptoms of bloating, abdominal pain and diarrhoea, or alternating diarrhoea and constipation. Systemically, gut toxins and pathogens can be absorbed into the blood stream giving rise to food intolerances, liver toxicity, auto-immune conditions and immune system deficiency. As the conversion of food to energy is compromised, fatigue and metabolic depression can develop.

Repairing the leaky gut and normalizing the gut health can produce far reaching health benefits.

14) The Liver

Gastro-intestinal health problems offer enough material for a complete book. Sufficient to say that the liver plays a major role in stress handling, immune support and elimination of gut toxins. It is the chief organ for detoxifying gut toxins which pass into the circulation. As I have already explained the bulk of T_4 to T_3 conversion occurs in the liver. Therefore toxaemia as a result of a leaky gut or poor absorption can compromise the liver's health and depress the thyroid's efficiency.

15) Heredity

When I am consulted by a patient with a suspected low grade hypothyroid, I always ask for information on their family health. Dr Stephen E. Langer in his book *Solved the Riddle of Illness* states that, 'Heredity is also an important factor'. He comments, however, that the increasing population of persons with hypothyroidism is not entirely a result of heredity[4]. The discovery of antibiotics has resulted in fewer thyroid patients dying with infections. The infant mortality rate at the turn of the century was around 50 per cent. The survivors were those who were able to resist infectious diseases. (This group did not usually include hypothyroid patients.) So in common with the increased incidence of diabetes since the discovery of insulin, thyroid conditions have increased since the use of life-saving antibiotics. There is a certain irony in a situation where lives are saved allowing for increased procreation and the incidence of hereditary disorders to escalate.

In his classic book *The Thyroid Gland* published in 1917, Robert McCarrison observed. 'There is a marked hereditary tendency or family predisposition to the disease. Sub-thyroidism in the mother is a common cause of sub-thyroidism in the child'.[5]

Research has shown that women with underactive thyroids are

four times more likely to have children with low IQ's than healthy mothers' children.

16) Tobacco

Tobacco contains a substance named thyocyanide. This is a powerful inhibitor of thyroid function, being identified as early as 1854. This adverse influence is particularly noted when iodine is deficient.

17) Fluoridation of Water

Iodine which is essential for the health of the thyroid can be displaced by fluoride and the gland will become depressed and underactive. Fluoride can also disturb the pituitary gland. It has been demonstrated that when animals are given fluoridated water (equivalent to human drinking-water fluoridation), their output of thyroid hormones is reduced. Surely a good case for drinking bottled mineral water.

18) Essential Fatty (EFAs) Acid Deficiency

Dr Robert Atkins has made a very important statement in his new book, 'What is becoming inescapably clear is that the essential fatty acids are collectively the number one missing nutrient in the American diet'[6].

'Essential' in this context means that the body cannot synthesize EFAs so they need to be obtained from foods or supplements.

The fatty acids are vitamin-like fats which perform many functions in the human body and are found in every membrane and cell in the body. Sometimes called 'vitamin F', they also act as precursors for prostaglandins. The prostaglandins or PGs are vital short-lived regulators which play a role in virtually every aspect of our metabolic processes.

The links between EFAs and thyroid function have yet to be clearly established. However evidence suggests that they can help prevent auto-immune diseases including SLE (Lupus), rheumatoid arthritis and psoriasis. They can also reduce the risk of auto-immune thyroidisis, and are prescribed for many conditions including arthritis, immune malfunction, skin health, pre-menstrual syndrome, diabetes, cancer, bowel conditions, fatigue and blood fat and heart disorders.

Unlike saturated fats which are solid at room temperature and processed mainly from animal products, the EFAs are usually in liquid form and their main sources are plants and fish.

Readers may be confused over the terms omega-3 and omega-6 which are used to classify some of the EFAs. The plan below shows the fat family members and their chief dietary sources.

FATS

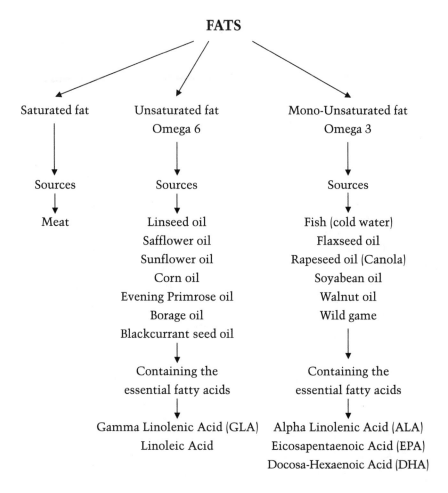

The 'omega' number depends on the positioning of double bonds in the molecular structure of the fatty acids. A subgroup, sometimes called the omega-9 group, can be found in nuts, olives and avocados.

The omega-9 oils from these foods are usually used for cooking, and feature widely in the Eastern Mediterranean diet. This region owes its low heart disease record to a diet rich in complex carbohydrates, fish, olives, nuts, game and antioxidant rich fresh fruits and vegetables.

Many doctors and researchers believe that the Western diet contains too high a percentage of omega-6 fatty acids in relation to the omega 3 group.

Accessibility, cost and the processing methods of the omega-3s all play their part in the imbalance between these essential fats. Diets which contain a high ratio of the omega-6 group have been linked to cancer promotion, low immune function, asthma, inflammatory joint conditions (e.g. rheumatoid arthritis and lupus) and raised blood pressure.

> This is not meant as a warning and readers will think that there is a paradox here. I am pointing a finger at the omega-6 fatty acids as a potential cause of the increased incidence of cancer, arthritis, chronic fatigue and heart disease in the UK and the USA, and yet omega-6s are essential for our health. To convert gamma linolenic acid (GLA) to the vital prostaglandin E1 a 'clear run' is needed along the metabolic pathway. The presence of vitamin B_3 and vitamin C are needed and vitamin E is also essential to prevent oxidation of the oil. A specific enzyme called delta-6-desaturase (D6D) is also essential before the omega-6s can become GLAs, and hypothyroidism, diabetes and immune breakdown can all reduce the availability of D6D. Only natural, unadulterated oil converts directly to GLA. Many dietary factors can 'block' the conversion. These include alcohol, saturated fats and low levels of magnesium, zinc and vitamin C.

As will be discussed in chapter 10 dealing with treatment, synergistic supplements need to be considered when taking any of the EFAs. The containers used to store oil should never be clear glass or plastic, as light can damage the oils. Organic, first-pressed oil is also to be preferred.

In spite of the popularity of evening primrose oil in the United Kingdom, borage oil contains four times more EFAs. Unfortunately, borage oil is not widely available on supermarket shelves and is therefore a costly supplement.

I always encourage my patients where possible to obtain their EFAs through their food. Particularly by eating fish regularly and using good quality oils. However supplementation is sometimes necessary to speed up recovery.

Summary

The length of this appendix serves to highlight the great number and diversity of factors that can contribute to mild hypothyroidism. Many of these causes can be uncovered by thorough case-history taking and laboratory testing. However, I am sure that my colleagues will agree with me when I say that mild hypothyroidism rarely develops as a result of a single cause.

Glossary

Adrenaline	Also known as epinephrine. A hormone produced by the adrenal glands to facilitate sudden physical activity in an emergency, and to raise the blood sugar level.
Adrenal Glands	Two glands, located adjacent to the top of each kidney. Consisting of two portions, the cortex and the medulla. The cortex secretes cortisol (hydrocortisone), cortisone and adrenal androgens. The androgens serve as precursors to testosterone and oestrogens. The medulla secretes adrenaline (epinephrine) and nor-adrenaline (norepinephrine).
Agoraphobia	An anxiety disorder caused by fear of open spaces and crowded public places.
Alzheimer's Disease	Premature senility, symptoms include confusion, memory failure, speech and movement difficulties, restlessness, loss of intelligence and judgement.
Amenorrhoea	The absence of menstruation.

Anaemia	A low level of blood haemoglobin. Causes include a reduction in red cell production, increased red cell destruction or blood loss. Classification is determined by the haemoglobin level and by the red cell size. There exist more than 90 different named anaemias, defined usually by their cause.
Anorexia	Condition caused by a prolonged refusal to eat and characterized by emaciation, amenorrhoea, neurosis and fear of obesity. Self induced vomiting and starvation can require hospitalization. Usually found in young women.
Arthritis	Inflammation of joints, usually with pain and swelling.
Atheroma	An abnormal build up of fat in an arterial wall.
Atherosclerosis	A disorder of the arteries involving a thickening of the blood vessel walls and a subsequent narrowing of the arteries, resulting in reduced blood flow. Atherosclerosis is a type of arteriosclerosis.
Attention Deficit Disorder (ADD)	A disorder with learning and behavioural disabilities in children and adolescents. Symptoms include hyperactivity, short attention span, and speech and memory problems. More common in boys than girls.
Autism	Mental disorder characterized by poor communication skills, delusions, hallucinations and a withdrawal from reality. Patients are usually totally self-centered.
Autoimmune Disease	Disorder caused as a result of the immune response being directed against the body's own tissues. SLE (lupus) and rheumatoid arthritis have been classified as auto-immune diseases. The precise cause is not known.

Autonomic Nervous System	A part of the nervous system that regulates non-voluntary functions, including the heart muscle, the intestines and the endocrine glands. It divides into the sympathetic and the parasympathetic branches.
Barnes Temperature Test	A thyroid function test designed by Dr Broda Barnes. This basal temperature test involves a minimum of three on-waking underarm temperature checks. Low levels can be found in mild hypothyroidism, and other disorders.
Basal Temperature	The temperature taken in the morning after sleep and before any activity, including moving, talking, eating, drinking or smoking.
Beta carotene	A red or orange pro-vitamin that is converted in the body to vitamin A.
Brown Fat	A type of fat that surrounds the kidneys, heart and adrenal glands. It is also found around the neck and upper spine. Its two chief functions are temperature and weight control. Brown fat accounts for around 10 per cent of the body's fat and it decreases with age.
Bulimia	Insatiable food craving. The binges are often followed by abdominal pain and self-induced vomiting. Unlike anorexia, weight loss does not always occur.
Bursitis	Inflammation of the bursa, the connective tissue structure that surrounds a joint. Bursitis can be caused by arthritis, infection, injury, excessive exercise or trauma e.g. housemaid's knee.
Calcitonin	A hormone produced by the thyroid. Its function is to reduce the level of calcium in the blood.
Candidiasis	An infection caused by candida albicans. Symptoms can include nappy (diaper) rash, vaginitis, thrush (vaginal or oral) and pruritus.

Carpal Tunnel	A conduit in the wrist enclosing the median nerve and the flexor tendons. Compression of the median nerve is termed carpal tunnel syndrome.
Cellulitis	Inflammation of the skin and/or nearby tissue. Symptoms include redness, heat, swelling and pain. Usually caused by an infection and /or poor circulation.
Cholesterol	A fat soluble substance occurring in animal fats, oils and egg yolks. Found in the bile, blood, brain tissue, liver, kidneys, adrenal glands and nerves. Precursor of steroid and sex hormones including cortisol, cortisone, DHEA, progesterone, oestrogen and testosterone. Cholesterol can crystallize in the gall bladder to form gall stones. Only 40 per cent of the total cholesterol is dietary, the remaining 60 per cent being produced by the liver.
Crohn's Disease	Inflammatory disease of the intestines. Scarring and thickening of the bowel wall can occur, with abscesses and diarrhoea. Also called regional enteritis.
Corticosteroids	The hormones associated with the adrenal cortex. Grouped as glucocorticoids (cortisol and corticosterone) and mineralocorticoids (aldosterone). Functions include control or influence of carbohydrate and protein metabolism, fluid balance, circulation system, skeletal muscles, kidneys and other organs.
Cortisol (Hydrocortisone)	A steroid hormone produced by the adrenal cortex. Functions include glucose metabolism and protein and fat regulation. It assists in regulation of the immune system.

Cortisone	A steroid hormone, involved in carbohydrate and protein regulation. It can be converted into cortisol. However, most of the cortisone found in the body is formed from cortisol by reversible reaction.
Cretinism	Severe congenital hypothyroidism.
Cysititis	Inflammation of the bladder. Symptoms include pain, frequency and blood in the urine. Although usually caused by bacterial infection, there are over eighteen variations of cystitis.
Dementia	A progressive mental disorder with personality disintegration, confusion, disorientation, poor judgement and memory. Causes include hyperthyroidism, drug abuse, Alzheimer's disease, brain tumour etc.
Desiccated Thyroid	Dried animal thyroid. Perhaps the oldest form of specific thyroid therapy, now largely replaced by raw glandular therapy.
DHEA (Dehydroepiandrosterone)	A 'mother' hormone, made from cholesterol and released by the adrenal glands. The precursor hormone of many steroid and sex hormones.
Dupuytren's Contracture	A progressive, usually painless, thickening and tightening of the tissues of the palm. The little and ring fingers are mainly affected.
Dysmenorrhoea	Painful periods, usually causing abdominal and spinal pain.
ELISA Test (Enzyme-Linked Immunosorbent Assay)	A blood test that can be used to identify food sensitivities. Food specific antibodies (IgG's) are measured when the blood contacts a panel of foods.
Endocrine Axis	Term used to describe the interlinked glands including the pituitary, thyroid and adrenal glands.

Erysipelas	An infectious skin disease, symptoms include swelling, blistering, redness, pain and fever.
ESR (Erythrocyte Sedimentation Rate)	The rate at which red cells settle in a tube of unclotted blood. Raised levels are non-specific, indicating the presence of inflammation. Particularly valuable in the diagnosis and monitoring in certain rheumatic diseases.
EFAs (Essential Fatty Acids)	These are fatty acids that cannot be synthesized by human metabolism and must therefore be obtained via food and drink.
Endocrine System	A network of glands that secrete hormones directly into the bloodstream. These include the pituitary, the thyroid, the adrenals, and the pineal gland etc.
Electrocardiogram (ECG)	A record of the electric activity of the heart muscle.
Enzyme	An enzyme is a protein substance that catalyses chemical reactions of various substances without itself being destroyed or altered. Although many enzyme reactions occur within cells, digestive enzymes operate outside the cells in the digestive tract.
Euthyroid	Describes a normal thyroid gland.
Ferritin	An iron compound stored in the liver, spleen and bone marrow. The ferritin level in the blood is seen as a useful indicator of the body's iron stores.
Fibromyalgia	A form of muscular rheumatism. Symptoms include musculo-skeletal aching and stiffness, fatigue and insomnia.
Fibrositis	See Fibromyalgia.
Gastrogram	A gastric function test designed to assess gastric acid production (pH), pancreatic enzyme levels and stomach emptying speed.

Geopathic Stress	Earth energy pathways or fields can be interfered with or blocked by railway and telegraph lines and overhead power lines. The pylons are seen to 'steal' the energy flow. Geopathic stress may be located by dowsing or by measuring air conductivity and background ionizing radiation levels.
Glucose Tolerance Factor	A complex comprising chromium, niacin (vitamin B³) and the amino acids glycine, glutamic acid and cysteine. The GTF is involved in the glucose–insulin balance.
Glucose Tolerance Test (GTT)	A two, five or six hour test involving frequent blood glucose measurements after the ingestion of 50–100gm of soluble glucose. The GTT is used as an aid to the diagnosis of diabetes and hypoglycaemia.
Glycogen	The chief carbohydrate stored in animal cells. It is formed from glucose and stored mainly in the liver and muscles. It can be converted back into glucose and released into the circulation when needed.
Goitre (Goiter)	Swelling in the neck caused by an enlarged thyroid gland. A goitre can be caused by hyperthyroidism, hypothyroidism and euthy-roidism.
Graves' Disease (Exophthalmic Goitre or Thyrotoxicosis)	Hyperthyroidism with goitre and exophthalmus (abnormal protrusion of the eyeballs).
Haemoglobin (Hb)	A protein–iron compound in the blood, that carries oxygen to the cells from the lungs and carbon dioxide away from the cells to the lungs.
Haemosiderin	An iron-rich pigment used as iron storage.
Hashimoto's Thyroiditis	Auto-immune hypothyroidism usually with a goitre.

Heliobactor Pylori	A bacterial infection that can cause gastritis and stomach ulcers. Usually treated with specific antibiotics.
Hormone Replacement Therapy (HRT)	Replacement of female hormones (oestrogen and/or progesterone). Although chiefly prescribed during and after menopause or hysterectomy, HRT is also prescribed for depression, osteoporosis, arthritis, Alzheimer's disease, low sex drive and pre-menstrual syndrome.
Hydrocortisone	See Cortisol.
Hyperinsulinism	Inappropriately high levels of insulin in the blood. Also defined as insulin resistance. Elevated blood insulin leads to calories being converted to fat instead of energy. Hypoglycaemia can also result from insulin excess.
Hyperthyroidism	Hyperactivity of the thyroid gland. This can accelerate all the metabolic processes of the body.
Hyperventilation	An excessive rate of breathing, leading to excessive oxygen intake and carbon dioxide elimination. This can lead to dizzyness, fainting, numbness of the fingers and toes and panic attacks. The many causes include hyperthyroidism, asthma, excessive exercising, meningitis, drug side effects and acute anxiety and fear.
Hypoglycaemia	Inappropriate low level of blood glucose. Usually caused by adrenal hypofunction or an insulin excess (as in poor diabetes control or hyperinsulinism).
Hypothyroidism	Underactivity of the thyroid gland.
Impetigo	A contagious (contact only) bacterial skin infection. Usually seen in children and located on the face, around the nose and mouth. Treatment includes antibiotic therapy.

Intermittent Claudication	Symptoms of pain, cramping and weakness in the legs that occur with use and improve with rest. The symptoms become progressively worse with walking. Caused by deficient blood supply in the legs, leading to reduced oxygen to the muscles.
IBS (Irritable Bowel Syndrome)	Also called mucous colitis, functional bowel syndrome or spastic colon. Symptoms include abdominal pain and fullness, intestinal wind and bowel disturbances.
Kwashiorkor (Infantile Pellagra)	Severe protein deficiency, usually seen in children. Symptoms include retarded growth, skin changes, mental apathy and anaemia. Mainly occurs in the tropics.
Kyphosis	An abnormal condition of the thoracic spine causing a 'hunchback' appearance. Severe forms can be caused by rickets, tuberculosis and ankylosing spondylitis. Mild kyphosis can be treated with osteopathy or chiropractic and correct dietary management.
Leaky Gut Syndrome	Increased gut permeability. This can allow the leakage of toxic substances from the gut into the blood stream. Chronic gut inflammation caused by candida albicans and other parasites can cause a leaky gut.
Libido	The sex drive or energy.
Lupus (SLE or Systemic Lupus Erythematous)	A chronic inflammatory auto-immune disease affecting many body systems.
Lyme Disease (Lyme Arthritis)	An acute recurrent inflammatory infection following a bite from a tick from a deer or wild pony or other animal. Named after Lyme in Connecticut USA where the condition was first described.

Malabsorption	Poor assimilation of nutrients including minerals, and fat soluble vitamins through the gastrointestinal tract or gut. This can occur in many disorders including diarrhoea, gluten sensitivity (coeliac disease), malnutrition, Crohn's disease, stomach surgery etc.
Ménière's Disease or Syndrome	Chronic disease of the middle ear, characterized by vertigo, hearing loss, tinnitus, nausea, vomiting and sweating. Attacks may last from a few minutes to several hours. Causes include infection and trauma.
Menorrhagia	Abnormally heavy or prolonged menstrual periods. The excessive blood loss can lead to anaemia. (A patient suffering from menorrhagia can lose iron equivalent to 4–6 weeks' dietary iron intake).
Myalgic Encephalomyelitis	A chronic illness with symptoms of fatigue, muscle–joint pain, depression and immune deficiency. The term ME is being replaced by chronic fatigue syndrome (CFS). Many doctors consider that ME is psychological in origin and prescribe antidepressant drugs and stress counselling.
Myxoedema	A severe form of hypothyroidism.
Naturopathy	A treatment system which recognises the human body possesses self-curative properties which resist disease. Naturopathic medicine may include hydrotherapy, dietetics, exercise and manipulation. Naturopaths often make use of other auxiliary techniques, including acupuncture, homoeopathy and herbalism.
Omega-3, -6, and -9	The essential fatty acids. The numbers refer to the position of the final

double bond carbon atoms at the methyl or 'omega' end of the molecules.

Osgood-Schlatter Disease — Knee inflammation usually seen in teenage boys. Involves swelling below the knee-cap with pain and inflammation. Caused by low mineral status and poor diet, coupled with rapid growth rate and excessive exercise.

Osteoporosis — Abnormal reduction in bone mass, leading to fractures from slight strain. Causes can include post-menopausal calcium depletion, lack of exercise in the elderly, poor diet and steroid therapy and thyroid or parathyroid disease.

Paraesthesia (Pins and Needles) — Generally describes a feeling of numbness, prickling, burning or tingling, usually in the hands or feet.

Parathyroid Glands — Several small glands (usually four in number), attached to the thyroid gland. They secrete the parathyroid hormone which aids regulation of calcium metabolism.

Pernicious Anaemia — Anaemia caused by lack of the intrinsic factor that is essential for the efficient absorption of vitamin B^{12}.

Perimenopause (Premenopause) — The phase before a woman's full menopause, when ovarian hormone production is reducing. Symptoms can begin as early as 35 years old and last for up to 15 years. The effects can include depression, muscle–joint problems, fatigue, headaches, insomnia, mood swings, osteoporosis, weight gain and loss of sex drive.

pH — Abbreviation for 'potential hydrogen'. A scale that represents the relative alkalinity or acidity of a solution. Neutral is 7.0, below 7.0 is acid and above 7.0 is alkaline. The pH value shows the relative hydrogen concentration of hydrogen atoms in a solution.

Phytoestrogens	Plant oestrogens, chiefly found in soya beans. These weak oestrogens are common in Asian and vegetarian diets and are seen by many doctors and health workers as the chief reason for low levels of menstrual and menopausal symptoms in Japanese women.
Pituitary Gland	A vital endocrine gland in the skull, responsible for control of the other endocrine glands e.g. adrenals, thyroid, pituitary and ovaries.
PMS (Pre-Menstrual Syndrome)	A group of symptoms that occur before menstruation. These can include fluid retention, hypoglycaemia, mood changes and fatigue.
Polymyalgia Rheumatica (Temporal Arteritis)	An auto-immune rheumatic disease, usually of the elderly. Symptoms can include arteritis (inflammation of the blood vessels), and severe muscle–joint stiffness following rest. Usually treated with steroid hormones. Total remission can occur after 12–18 months.
Prediabetes	Mild, first stage diabetes. Usually controlled by diet alone.
Pregnenolone	Sometimes called the 'mother' hormone, because other hormones including DHEA, oestrogen, testosterone, cortisol and proges-terone are synthesized from pregnenolone. An adrenal steroid hormone, it is prescribed for depression and rheumatic symptoms.
Raynaud's Phenomena	Reduced blood flow to the fingers, toes, ears and nose. Symptoms include whiteness followed by cyanosis (bluish discolouration) and pain. Causes include rheumatoid arthritis, lupus, neck and upper spinal pressure, drug side effects, malnutrition, hyperthyroidism, injury and high blood pressure. If severe, gangrene can develop.

RSI (Repetitive Strain Injury)	Pain and stiffness in the hands, arms, neck, shoulders or back. Usually caused by the repetitive use of particular muscles and joints, which in itself is not painful but over a long period of use can become severely painful. Often occupational and currently the subject of many work related injury claims.
Rheumatism	A term used to describe a large group of conditions that involve inflammation, pain and stiffness of joints, ligaments and muscles. These include arthritis, gout, lupus and spondylitis.
SAD Syndrome (Seasonal Affective Disorder)	A mood disorder triggered by season change. It involves a poor response to light loss during the winter months. Many workers consider that the pineal gland and the melatonin that is secreted by the pineal gland is the key to SAD treatment and control.
Scoliosis	Lateral spinal curvature. More than 16 types have been identified, and defined according to their cause.
SLE	see Lupus.
Sleep Apnoea	An absence of spontaneous breathing, occurring during sleep. The attacks are usually transient and brief.
Tendonitis (Tendinitis)	Inflammation of a tendon. Usually resulting from strain.
Tendosynovitis (Tenosynovitis)	Inflammation of a tendon sheath. Causes can include strain, poor circulation, raised blood cholesterol, rheumatoid arthritis, gout and calcium deposits.
Tetany	A condition caused by a disorder of calcium metabolism and vitamin D deficiency. An underactive parathyroid gland or taking an excess of alkaline salts can also cause the

	symptoms. These include cramp, convulsions, muscle twitching and involuntary flexion of the wrists and ankles.
Tinnitus	Noises in the ears including buzzing, ringing, singing etc. Very common and when severe, very distressing. Causes can include excessive noise (e.g. pop concerts, or personal stereos etc.), wax in the ears, catarrh, high and low blood pressure, anaemia, vertigo, drug side effects, bleeding from the ear, Ménière's disease, ear diseases and cervical disc lesions.
Thyroxine (T₄)	The chief thyroid hormone.
Triiodothyronine (T₃)	The most active thyroid hormone metabolized from thyroxine in the peripheral tissue.
TRH (Thyrotropin Releasing Hormone)	A hormone released from the hypothalamus in the brain to stimulate the release of the pituitary hormone thyrotropin (TSH).
TSH (Thyroid Stimulating Hormone) or Thyrotropin	A pituitary hormone that controls the release of the thyroid hormones. It is measured in the blood to assess the thyroid balance.
Uric Acid	A substance in the blood resulting from protein metabolism and excreted through the bladder. When in excess, it forms into crystals causing gout. An excess of uric acid in the kidneys can give rise to the formation of kidney stones.
Vitiligo	A benign skin disease of unknown cause. Thought to be an auto-imune condition. Symptoms include loss of skin pigment in patches. The adrenal and thyroid glands and the pancreas may be involved.
Xanthelasma	Small yellow, fatty spots around the corners of the upper and lower eyelids. Causes can include excessive blood fats and diabetes.

Resources

Support Groups

American Foundation of Thyroid Patients
P O Box 820195
Houston
TX 77282-0195
(281) 496-4460

Australian Thyroid Foundation
P O Box 186
Westmead NSW 2145
Australia
61-2-9890-6962

British Thyroid Foundation
P O Box 97
Clifford
Wetherby
West Yorkshire
LS23 6XD

For further information please send
a large stamped addressed envelope.

Thyroid Foundation of America Inc.
40 Parkman Street
Boston
MA 02114-2698
1-888-996-4460

Thyroid Eye Disease Association
34 Fore Street
Chudleigh
Devon
TQ13 0HX

The author may be contacted at:
Ridge Cottage
29 Ferncroft Road
Bournemouth
Dorset
BH10 6BY
(Please enclose a stamped self-addressed envelope).
www.martin–budd.com
e-mail: mlb@martin–budd.com

Supplement Suppliers

ABCO Laboratories
2450 S Watney Way
(Solano Business Part)
Fairfield
CA 94533
USA

Nutri West
P O Box 950
Douglas
Wyoming
WY 82633
USA

Nutri Ltd
Buxton Road
New Mills
High Peak
SK22 3JU

Further Reading

Aren, Dr Ridha. *The Thyroid Solution*

Atkins, Dr Robert C. *Dr Atkins' Vita-Nutrient Solution*, Simon and Schuster

Barnes, Broda. *Hypothyroidism – The Unsuspected Illness*, Harper and Row

Budd, Martin L. *Low Blood Sugar*, London, Thorsons

Chaitow, Leon. *Fibromyalgia and Muscle Pain*, London, Thorsons

Chaitow, Leon. *The Beat Fatigue Workbook*, London, Thorsons

Einzig, Hetty and Cannon, Geoffrey. *Dieting Makes You Fat*, Sphere

Ford, Gillian. *Listening to Your Hormones*, Prima Publishing

Gittleman, A. L. *Eat Fat – Lose Weight*, Keats

McCarrison, Robert. *The Thyroid Gland*, Baillière, Tindall and Cox (now out of print)

McConnell, Carol and Malcolm. *The Mediterranean Diet*, Bodley Head

Newman Turner, Roger. *Naturopathic Medicine*, London, Thorsons

Rogerson and Colman. *The Super Hormone Promise*, Avon Books

Rosenthal, M. Sara. *The Thyroid Source Book*, Lowell House

Scheer, James and Langer, Stephen. *Solved the Riddle of Illness*, Keats

Tunbridge and Bayliss. *Thyroid Disease – The Facts*, Oxford University Press

Westcott, Patsy. *Thyroid Problems*, London, Thorsons

Williams, Xandra. *Fatigue*, Cedar

Wilson, E. Denis. *Wilson's Syndrome*, Cornerstone Publishing

References

Chapter 2

1 Leon Chaitow, *Fibromyalgia and Muscle Pain* (London, Thorsons, 1998)

Chapter 3

1 Geoffrey Cannon, *Dieting Makes You Fat* (Sphere Books Ltd, 1984)
2 Jeffrey Bland, *Your Personal Health Programme* (London, Thorsons, 1993)
   Jeffrey Bland, *Clinical Nutrition* (The Institute for Functional Medicine, 1999)
3+4 Geoffrey Cannon, *Dieting Makes You Fat* (Sphere Books Ltd, 1984)

Chapter 4

1 'Diagnostic and Statistical Manual of Mental Disorders' *DSM-111* (The American Psychiatric Association)
2 Ridha Arem, *The Thyroid Solution* (Ballantine Books, 1999)
3 Leon Chaitow, *The Beat Fat Workbook* (London, Thorsons, 1988)

Chapter 5

1   John R. Lee, *Natural Progesterone, The Multiple Roles of a Remarkable Hormone* (BLL Publications, 1994)
2   G. E. Abraham, 'Nutritional Factors in the Aetiology of the Premenstrual Tension Syndromes', *J. Repro. Med, 1983.28. : 446-464*
3   H. Gardner-Hill and J. F. Smith, *Journal of Obst and Gynae. Brit Emp. 34: 701* (1927)
4   Broda O. Barnes, 'The Treatment of Menstrual Disorders in General Practice', *Arizona Medicine 6:33* (1949)
5   J. C. Scott and E. Mussey 'Menstrual Patterns in Myxedema', *American Journal Obst and Gynea* (September 1964)

Chapter 6

1   W.M. Ord 'On Mxoedema, A Term Proposed to be Applied to an Essential Condition in the Cretinoid Infection Occasionally Observed in Middle-Aged Women' *Trans. Med-Churg Soc. 60-61: 57-78* (1877-78)
2   V. Horsley 'The Thyroid Gland' *British Medical Journal 1:211 (1885)*
3   Robert McCarrison, *The Thyroid Gland in Health and Disease*, (Baillere, Tindall and Cox) OOP
4   L.T. Swain 'Chronic Arthritis' *J.A.M.A 93:259* (1929)
5   P.N. Golding, 'Hypothyroidism Presenting with Musculo-Skeletal Symptoms', *An. Rheum. Dis. 29:10* (1970)
6   Krupsky, Flatau, Yarom and Resnitzky, 'Musculoskeletal Symptoms as a Presenting Sign of a Long-Standing Hypothyroidism', *Israel Journal of Medical Sciences 23* (1976)
7   Broda O. Barnes, *Hypothyroidism – The Unsuspected Illness* (Harper and Row, 1976)

Chapter 7

1   Stephen E. Langer, *Solved the Riddle of Illness* (Keats Publications, 1984)
2   A. Lidsky and K. Kottman, 'Influence of Thyroids on Blood Clotting' *Zeitschrift Klin Medicin 71:344* (1911)

Chapter 8

1   Broda O. Barnes, *Hypothyroidism – The Unsuspected Illness* (Harper and Row, 1976)
2   C. D. Eaton, 'Coexistence of Hypothyroidism with Diabetes Mellitus' *Journal Michigan Medical Society 53:101* (1954)
3   O. Schaefer, 'Glucose Tolerance Testing in Canadian Eskimos: A Preliminary Report and a Hypothesis' *Canadian Medical Journal 99:252* (1968)
4   M. B. Lurie, *Resistance to Tuberculosis: Experimental Studies in Native and Acquired Defensive Mechanisms* (Cambridge, Mass. Harvard University Press, 1964)

Chapter 9

1   Broda O. Barnes, *Hypothyroidism – The Unsuspected Illness* (Harper and Row, 1976)
2   E. Denis Wilson, *Wilson's Syndrome* (Orlando, USA, Cornerstone Publications, 1996)
3   G. Luden, 'Studies on Cholesterol: V. The Blood Cholesterol in Malignant Disease and the Effect of Radium on the Blood Cholesterol, Collected Papers', *Mayo Clinic Vol 10*, (Philadelphia, W.B. Saunders, 1918)
4   J. J. Westra and M. M. Kunde, ' Blood Cholesterol in Experimental Hypo and Hyperthyroidism' *Proc. Soc. Exper. Biol and Med. 29:677* (1932)
5   J. P. Simmonds and O. E. Helper 'Fat Tolerance in Experimental Hyperthyroidism' *J.A.M.A. 98:283* (1932)

6 Lewis M. Hurxtham, 'Blood Cholesterol and Thyroid Disease' *Archives Internal Medicine Vol 53: 762-781* (1934)

7 Broda O. Barnes, *Hypothyroidism – The Unsuspected Illness* (Harper and Row, 1976)

Chapter 10

1 Roger Newman-Turner, *Naturopathic Medicine* (London, Thorsons, 1985) OOP

2 Leon Chaitow, *The Raw Materials of Health,* (London, Thorsons, 1989)

3 Martin Budd, *Diets to Help Migraine* (London, Thorsons, 1997) OOP

4 P. L. MacKendrick and V. M. Scramuzza, *The Ancient World* (New York, Holt, Reinhart and Winston, 1958)

Appendix

1 Gordon R. B. Skinner et al, 'Thyroxine Should be Tried in Clinical Hypothyroid but Biochemically Euthyroid Patients' *(Letters) B.M.J. Vol 214* (1997)

2 I.W. Jennings, *Vitamins in Endocrine Metabolism,* (Springfield, IL, C. C. Thomas, 1970

3 Ridha Arem, *The Thyroid Solution* (Ballantine Books, 1999)

4 R. Bruce Gillie, 'Endemic Goitre' *Scientific American* (June 1971)

5 Stephen E. Langer, *Solved the Riddle of Illness* (Keats Publications, 1984)

6 R. MacHarrison, *The Thyroid Gland* (London, Bailliere, Tindall and Cox, 1917) OOP

7 Robert C. Atkins, *Dr Atkins' Vita-Nutrient Solution* (Fireside Books, 1999)

Index